Change Your Mind About Tinnitus

Transforming the Way You Think To Help Control the Ringing in Your Ears

Paul D'Arezzo, M.D.

Marcellina Mountain Press

Disclaimer:

This book contains only the opinions and ideas of the author. It is not a substitute for medical treatment, and it is recommended that all those with tinnitus receive a thorough work-up by a medical professional prior to using the methods in this book. The author makes no claims and takes no responsibility for the results any given individual may obtain by following the prescribed advice or exercises in this book.

Cover design by highrealmgraphics.com

ISBN: 978-0-9729079-2-7

Marcellina Mountain Press

Table of Contents

Introduction 1

1 - My Story 5

2 - The Facts About Tinnitus 15

3 - It's A Big Deal 27

4 - How This Book Works 37

5 - Our Bodies and Minds Are Adaptable 47

6 - Why? 49

7 - What Do You Believe? 53

8 - Can I Ask You A Question? 71

9 - The Power of Words 79

10 - Don't Give It Energy 85

11 - Interrupt It! 91

12 - Disrupting Our Negative Patterns 99

13 - Scrambling Things Up (Even More) 115

14 - Make It a Game 121

15 - Action Plan 125

16 - Final Thoughts 141

About the Author: 144

Introduction

I know how bad it is to suffer from tinnitus. I know how totally devastating it can feel and how it can turn your life completely upside down. After doing everything I could to find a solution to either stop or control my tinnitus with little or no results, I realized that if I were going to live with this, it would be up to me.

While there are a number of treatment options available for tinnitus and I suggest you try or use any or all of those in conjunction with this book, tinnitus is unique in that there is a decidedly mental component to it. We all intuitively sense that if we could only control our minds, then that would help control our tinnitus and the effect it has on our lives. We know there should be a way to use our minds, the way we think, so that our minds are our allies in our struggle with tinnitus regardless of which other methods we may choose to use.

This book is neither an in-depth review of the causes of tinnitus nor a compendium of all possible tinnitus treatments. There are no other products or services I am trying to sell. Rather, this book has a simple, albeit significant, goal. Its sole purpose is to give those suffering from tinnitus some different ways of thinking and simple mental techniques to put their minds solidly on their side in their encounter with tinnitus. For many people, this may be enough to break the hold tinnitus has on their lives.

While people may tell to use your mind to help control tinnitus, they usually don't actually tell you how. Think positive. Distract yourself. That's good advice, but only as far as it goes. This book goes into far more detail, giving you proven mental and physical strategies to use your mind to both markedly diminish the emotional effect tinnitus has on your life and to functionally decrease the amount of time you focus on it.

The methods in this book are what I used for my tinnitus, and they worked. They aren't what you may be used to or expect. You may expect something more sophisticated or cerebral particularly from an author who is a doctor. But our minds are simple and often child-like in the way they deal with things.

Unlike a treatment where you take a pill or have a surgical procedure, the methods in this book require your personal involvement. You have to do your part. You have to take an active role and participate in your own rescue. And even if some of it doesn't make sense right away, you need to trust me. From this point forward, things will only get better.

Am I some super-human being with mental capacities beyond yours? No. In fact, while I was writing this book, I had a few days when I was having a particularly bad time dealing with my tinnitus. I said to my wife, "How can I be writing a book dealing with tinnitus when I'm feeling bad myself?" She gave me that look she gives me. Then she said, "That is exactly *why* you should write it," adding that I was one hundred times better than I had been before. And she was right on both counts. Too often people write books and pretend or think they should have all the answers. I've written other books. I know the feeling. It's easy to be glib and say, "Do this and all your problems will be solved." This book isn't like that; this book is written by someone down in the trenches just like you.

I do guarantee, however, that after finishing this book that you will not think and feel the same way about your tinnitus as you did before, and that it will have less of a detrimental effect on your life.

I suggest you get a notebook before you read the rest of this book so that you can write things down. Write down the exercises I ask you to do, but also write down the insights you have while reading the book. I believe we all know more than we think: at some level, we all know or secretly suspect the way out.

Again, I truly know the suffering of tinnitus. I can't say that enough times. This is the book I wish I had when I developed tinnitus. My motivation in writing this book is that if I can help one person in some way not to feel as bad, not to feel overcome by their tinnitus even for a few moments, then this book has been a worthwhile endeavor.

So let's begin.

Chapter One

My Story

What's that noise? That's the way it started. I was studying in my office when I noticed a loud whining noise coming from my left. What's that? It sounded like a very shrill electrical hum, almost as if some loud electrical appliance was left running inside the house. Or an alarm or siren was wailing off in the distance at an incredibly high and persistent pitch. I naturally turned my head to locate where the wailing was coming from. It was coming from my left. But when I stood up and turned around in the room, the noise still seemed to be coming from my left. That's strange, I thought. I walked around the house. No appliances were running. Nothing was out of the ordinary. The noise was so loud, so high-pitched, and so disturbing.

I went outside. The loud ringing was out there too; again, no matter in which direction I turned it still came from my left. It was then that I realized that it was coming from inside my left ear itself.

It had come on relatively quickly—one minute I was studying in silence, the next minute a loud shrieking was filling the left side of my head and garnering all my attention.

At first, I somehow didn't think it was bad, or at least not terribly bad. Instinctively, I put my finger into my left ear and poked around. I yawned and stretched my jaw. The ringing felt like when one's ears don't decompress on an airplane flight or on an underwater dive. But none of the ways I manipulated my ear or mouth made the least difference. This certainly is loud and annoying I said to myself. But I also told myself that this was probably just some quirky thing that would go away in a few minutes. I thought my ear would somehow 'pop', and everything would be back to normal, and I'd think, "Jeez, that was weird," and it would be all over.

But it didn't go away, and almost as if on cue, it seemed to increase in intensity and became a now a *very* loud, high-pitched, all-consuming screeching in my left ear.

I knew a little about tinnitus, sometimes pronounced tin-ni-tus, sometimes pronounced tin-NI-tus—is this is what I had?

Cupping my hands over my ears, or covering the left side of my head with a pillow did nothing to alter the intense, high-pitched wail that had rapidly become a form of torture. In fact, over the next days, I would specifically look up on the Internet how people were able to survive torture, hoping to glean some trick or help in managing the terrible ringing. You have to abandon yourself to the fate that your pain might not ever end one article preached. Just what I needed.

The wailing was so loud. So unrelenting. So damned high-pitched. It rapidly began to drive me crazy. After enduring it for several hours, I lay on my bed with my knees pulled up into my chest, and my hands clasped over my ears, trying to endure the discomfort. I would breathe one breath at a time, feeling one breath come in and then go out. That's the way I felt I was surviving—one breath at a time. Someone help me, my brain called out. Someone please help me. But no one came and nothing changed. I was alone with this torture. I began to cry, a sort of hopeless, helpless, frustrated type of crying. I didn't know what I could do. I wanted to do something to make it stop but nothing I tried worked. I rapidly became at wit's end.

It might sound strange that so quickly over a number of hours I reached such a markedly deep state of despair, but it speaks in great part to the horror of this malady, or particularly of the severe form of tinnitus I was experiencing. It was and is that bad. I had never known something like this could be so frighteningly all consuming and unrelenting. I had always thought tinnitus was some sort of faint background buzzing perhaps like an insect humming off in the distance. But this was so loud and it had a glassy, particularly irritating quality to it. I couldn't imagine doing anything—eating, driving, reading, walking, or anything any of us associates with living a normal life—with this screeching in my ear.

A few hours later my wife returned from work. It was nice to have someone else—a caring soul—in the house with me now. By this time I was in a very bad state.

One analogy that came to my mind at that time was that this was akin to being in a prison cell with a deafening alarm blaring. But I thought to myself that people adjust to being around loud noises all day; why couldn't I just adjust to this, at least until I could get in to see a doctor. But this was somehow different or worse because the loud screaming came from *inside* my head itself (still only on the left). I couldn't distract myself from it because it was somehow part of me.

My wife helped. We both knew certain medications could cause tinnitus. I wasn't taking anything that could have caused it, but I decided to stop all my medications regardless in the hope that they were the cause.

We made our first tentative forays reading about tinnitus on the Internet, a singularly depressing experience. It certainly seemed that is what I had. People talked about having tinnitus for years and years and years. They spoke of the same torture that I had experienced for only a few hours. I rapidly decided I didn't want to read about tinnitus.

After another 48 hours, I was near suicidal. I can't imagine living like this I told myself. I don't want to live like this. I have no reason to live if I have to live like this. My family doctor examined my ears and found nothing abnormal. I had no history or signs of infection or head or neck trauma. I hadn't been exposed to any loud noises. He gave me a Xanax prescription and I was referred to get an audiogram and see an ear, nose and throat specialist (ENT) over the next few days. The audiogram showed some high-frequency hearing loss on my left where the ringing was. The following week—I was barely surviving day by day—I saw the ENT specialist who ordered an MRI (it was normal). As we get older, the hair cells in our inner ear sometimes begin to fail to respond as they should, and our brains create a sound, the ringing, to compensate for that loss of sound. That is what is going on. The sound is coming from your brain, the ENT doctor told me.

"Could you make me deaf in that ear and would it go away?" I asked him. I was that desperate.

"It wouldn't help. People have actually done that. Even if the nerve is cut, the ringing persists."

The only other thing he could offer was he said some people were helped by bioflavonoids and by acupuncture. I could try those things.

Day in and day out, the ringing persisted. Looking back I don't know how I survived. I did all the things people do to survive tinnitus. I played music and sounds to mask the ringing. I listened to waterfalls, showers, fans, endless rainstorms, vacuum cleaners, dryers, road noise, chimes, chirping birds, jungle noises, crickets, white noise, pink noise, brown noise, blue noise—yes, there are different colored noises you can listen to. I listened to yoga music, meditation music, music to study by. I listen to the droning sounds of brain wave music—theta waves—that are supposed to calm and realign the brain and psyche. I listened to all my favorite songs until I was sick of them. I used earphones and speakers. I adjusted the balance in various ways sending more or sometimes less sound to the ringing ear.

My only relative relief was taking a shower in the morning. The discordant sound of the shower and the splashing of the water against the tiles somewhat covered the ringing. I could actually think a few thoughts without the ringing intruding.

I read that if acupuncture is going to help, it ideally should be done right away. Over the next three weeks, I went to three different acupuncturists having a number of treatments with each. I remember looking down and seeing my arms pin-cushioned with slender needles while I listened to droning yoga-type music. One of the acupuncturists even gave me a homeopathic treatment consisting of small sesame-sized pills that I was to take without touching them with my hands, but rather was to pop them directly into my mouth from a plastic bag. Another of the acupuncturists advises me to increase the amount of starch in my diet. Despite what I did or tried, there was no change in my ringing.

Nights were still particularly bad. Some nights despite taking sleeping pills I'd wake up in the middle of the night with the screaming in my head. I'd try to cover it with noise, music or TV, but nothing was loud enough to cover it up. Sometimes I'd just lie on the floor in a ball. I didn't know how I could survive this.

I bought vitamins. Lots of vitamins. And minerals too. Zinc, magnesium, calcium, B-complex vitamins, stress complex vitamins, gingko (some studies show it helps), bioflavonoids, and lots of antioxidants.

At one health food store, I found myself staring at rows and rows of vitamins and supplements. I asked the young woman who seemed assigned to the area for help. She referred me to a massive compendium of natural treatments located in a nook off to one side. I looked up tinnitus. There was a long list of possible remedies including craniosacral manipulation, various roots, botanicals, herbs, extracts, and supplements. No one seemed sure what to do to cure this. I bought some more antioxidants and ginkgo supplements and went home.

I tried probiotics. Maybe my gut flora is deficient in some necessary bacilli, with my immune and hearing system being adversely affected. It's possible, I tell myself. I eat special yogurt with live cultures and drink kefir, which tastes like a buttermilk smoothie.

I take up juicing. Maybe I lack some essential nutrient that could only be found in fresh vegetable juices.

Temporomandibular joint (TMJ) dysfunction—maybe I have that, and that is causing the ringing. When I put my fingers in my ears and move my jaw, I do hear a slight clicking sound on the left where the ringing is. I copy down a series of TMJ exercises and practice them several times a day. One of called the goldfish; you hold your jaw and slowly open and close your mouth against resistance—like a goldfish.

I imagine some change, but I know there is no difference.

Maybe it has something to do with my Eustachian tubes, the tubes that equalize the pressure in the middle ear. I use nasal sprays. It doesn't help.

I listen to tinnitus hypnosis tapes online. If they have any benefit, it must be to in my deep subconscious, because the ringing remains as loud as ever.

Pills help. I have Xanax and two types of sleeping pills—Lunesta and Ambien. I try to avoid taking them but invariably almost every night I do. I like knowing I have the pills. I know I can usually fall asleep when it gets so bad. Despite the drugs, I don't sleep well or for very long. I don't dream. Invariably I reach a point every night where my body wants to sleep, but my brain, my head is too wired and alert from the ringing. The need for sleep and the ringing fight a pitched battle that goes on for hours unless I take a pill and eventually slog into a dreamless, non-restful sleep.

I am also drinking more wine than I should. At times, for an hour or so the wine drinking seems to mellow out the ringing. Most times when I watch TV, the ringing of the tinnitus overrides the sound of the TV. Sometimes with the wine, I can watch TV and can forget about or not hear the tinnitus for a few brief minutes.

Again, the night is the worst time for me. I dread the night. I fear the night. I hate the night. I fear how the ringing will become ever more high pitched and omnipresent. I don't like the thought that I will have to try to sleep tonight. I don't like the idea of fighting all over again tonight. At night I listen to music and sounds to try to mask the tinnitus. It doesn't help much.

In the morning when I wake up after finally falling asleep at three or four in the morning, I wake up half expecting, hoping that it—the ringing—will not be there. I hope. I pray. I imagine. But there, every morning it is, louder than ever. I wake up thinking I have to fight this another day. How can I do it? Waking up just means trying to survive. I can't do this. "Help me. Someone help me," I mouth my silent, endless prayer over and over.

The other thing is that other than my inconsistent sleep, there is no relief and no rest. With severe tinnitus like I was experiencing, you can't just lie down and rest and get away from it like you might from a sore leg or back. It is *always* there. In fact, when you lie down or try to rest, some perverse quality of it makes it grow louder. It becomes even more all consuming. You can't escape. You can't get away from it. There is no sanctuary.

Despite being a doctor, there is nothing special I can do differently than anyone else. I have no special magic or access to any treatments different than anyone else. There simply is no cure. There are strategies to deal with tinnitus: sound therapies, behavioral modification and cognitive therapies, hearing aids. I am open to trying any or all of them.

I read all the books I can find on tinnitus. At the medical library, I search through over eight hundred medical abstracts on tinnitus. The usual treatments are discussed. There are a few experimental treatments. Nothing is very encouraging

I see another audiologist who specializes in tinnitus. She tells me I won't get better and I have to accept it. She wants to sell me a hearing aid that will also mask the tinnitus. I tell her I will think about it.

I finally realize that although I may continue to try different things, dealing with tinnitus seems to fall squarely on my shoulders.

I want to survive. I want to get over this or learn to handle this. I just don't know how. For most things in my past, I just work harder. This is different. I don't know how to work harder to handle this. I certainly recognize there is a mental component to tinnitus—if I can control my mind, I can diminish the devastating effect tinnitus is having on me. That becomes my goal and the basis for this book.

If you can relate in any way to my story, then this book is for you.

Chapter Two

The Facts About Tinnitus

The U.S. Centers for Disease Control estimates that tinnitus in some form or another affects 15% of the country's population. That's roughly 20 million people, and of those, two million people are felt to have severe, debilitating tinnitus such that it drastically affects their lives.

What is tinnitus?

Tinnitus is the sensation of hearing sound in your ears when no external sound is present. These sounds can vary both in quality and intensity depending on the individual. They are commonly described as a ringing, buzzing, roaring, clicking, or hissing sound. For some, the sound is constant and unremitting. For others the sound may vary in pitch and loudness, and also may come and go.

Tinnitus is a generic word. It describes a symptom. If you tell someone that you have tinnitus it doesn't tell anyone about what may be causing it, just as if you told someone you have a headache it does not reveal what the cause of the headache may be.

What causes tinnitus?

The most common causes of tinnitus are—

Tinnitus in association with age-related hearing loss

As we get older, we generally lose our hearing starting at about age 60. Tinnitus often occurs in association with this. Damage to the tiny sensory hair cells in our inner ear simply due to aging and long-term exposure to noise is felt to be the cause of this. It is beyond the scope of this book to discuss this in detail but the noise, the ringing, from tinnitus is not coming from one's ear, but rather is produced by the brain itself in response to a deficit in certain frequencies of our hearing caused by the damage. Unfortunately, this common cause of tinnitus is generally not reversible.

Tumors of the head and neck or trauma to the head or neck

Masses inside the head or neck or trauma can damage or put pressure on the blood vessels and nerves that are involved with hearing and the delicate inner ear apparatus.

Exposure to loud noise

Loud noise, particularly if one is exposed to it for an extended period, can cause permanent damage to our ears and result in tinnitus. This could include such things as working around loud machinery, using firearms without proper ear protection, or exposure to loud music over long periods of time. Short-term exposure to loud noises such as at a rock concert can cause temporary tinnitus (and sometimes hearing loss), which usually resolves over hours or days.

Blockage or irritation to the external ear canal

The most common cause is the accumulation of excessive earwax, which can irritate the eardrum itself and cause tinnitus. This is most often readily reversible.

Middle ear abnormalities

Infections or anything associated with damage or irritation to the middle ear can cause tinnitus.

Abnormal growth of the bones of your middle ear (otosclerosis)

This is a rare inheritable disorder where the bones of your middle ear become fixed and unable to move and transmit sound as they should.

Meniere's Disease

Caused by abnormal inner ear fluid pressure, this disorder characteristically manifests with vertigo, tinnitus, and hearing loss. Specific treatments including medications and surgery may help.

Blood vessel (vascular) problems

Atherosclerosis—"hardening of the arteries"—can cause blood vessels to lose their elasticity and sometimes cause a pulsatile-type tinnitus. Similarly, other malformations of blood vessels can cause tinnitus, as can high blood pressure itself.

Temporomandibular Joint Problems (TMJ)

Misalignment and inflammation of our TMJ joints (where our mandible, or jaw bone, meets our skull) can cause tinnitus.

Medications

There are a number of medications that can cause tinnitus. The most common ones are the antibiotic "mycins" (polymyxin

B, erythromycin, vancomycin, and neomycin), certain diuretics ("water pills"), aspirin in high doses, quinine, cancer medications, and sometimes certain antidepressants. This is not an exhaustive list. When evaluating the cause of tinnitus, it is important to check with your doctor to see if any of your medications could be causing or contributing to your tinnitus.

Other causes

This above list of causes of tinnitus is not all-inclusive. That is why it is imperative that you receive a thorough evaluation for your tinnitus by a health professional, and by any additional specialist if indicated, and that you obtain any diagnostic tests that are required. Many of the above causes of tinnitus *are* readily treatable and can be cured.

That said, for many causes of tinnitus, health professionals can only make an educated guess on what is causing it based on all the evidence. For example, we can't directly see the tiny hair cells that may be damaged in the inner ear with tinnitus associated with aging, but putting a person's age together with associated hearing loss, a health professional can be reasonably certain that is the cause. Sometimes the exact cause of our tinnitus can be even more tenuous. No one may know for sure what caused it, and health providers may only be able to say, "We can't find anything reversible that is causing it."

How does tinnitus affect people?

This obviously varies with the given individual and with the intensity and persistence of the tinnitus. Tinnitus can often cause extreme stress and depression in many people, and total disruption of their normal life. It can make you extremely anxious, fearful, and irritable. It can affect your ability to concentrate, to remember things, and have a detrimental effect on one's job and home situation. It can change one's life dramatically. When it develops suddenly as in my case, it can be extremely disruptive and frightening.

At the same time, some people readily adjust to tinnitus and just somehow accept it.

For many, tinnitus is often particularly worse at night, when one is trying to go to sleep. Thus, it can often cause sleep disorders. As if that weren't enough, for others, it is often worse in the morning too upon awakening.

For some people, certain things make their tinnitus worse. Later in this book, I will help you discover and make a list of things that may tend to make your tinnitus worse. Avoiding these things or ameliorating their effect will be part of your overall strategy in dealing with tinnitus. Stress itself often makes tinnitus worse—any kind of stress. Obviously, this is a sort of Catch-22: If I didn't have this tinnitus, I wouldn't be stressed, now would I?

Hyperacusis, which refers to an increased sensitivity to normal sounds or certain frequencies of sounds, is often associated with tinnitus. Such things as a slamming car door, or the sounds inside a loud restaurant, can, along with being extremely irritating, cause an increase in one's tinnitus. For some exposure to loud noises can cause an exacerbation of their tinnitus which lasts for days.

What sort of medical evaluation is indicated for tinnitus?

In general, the medical evaluation of tinnitus involves the following.

First, be evaluated by your family physician. A thorough history and physical should help pinpoint possible causes of your tinnitus. Your doctor should be able to rule out many of the readily-reversible causes of tinnitus. These include such things as ear wax (cerumen) or foreign body blocking the ear canal, middle ear infection or abnormality, temporomandibular joint abnormality (TMJ), head or neck abnormalities, blood vessel problems, and medications.

Have an audiogram performed. This evaluates your hearing. Some hearing loss is often associated with certain types of tinnitus, and its presence helps in determining the likely cause of the tinnitus.

If necessary or recommended, see an ENT (ear, nose, and throat) specialist, or other specialist if indicated. If recommended, have an MRI (Magnetic Resonance Imaging) done. This is a special-type X-ray of your brain to rule out any tumors or other abnormalities that could be causing the problem.

If your tinnitus is reversible, no matter what its cause, it is better to get it treated as soon as possible. Again, don't skimp on having a thorough medical evaluation for your tinnitus.

Tinnitus, however, can be frustrating to health professionals too. Doctors and health professionals want to help people. They want to cure people. Unfortunately, with tinnitus after a certain point, they often don't have much if anything to offer. That's just the way it is. Tinnitus is one of those disorders where you have to take a certain amount of personal responsibility for it yourself. You have to be your own advocate in getting a thorough evaluation, in educating yourself, and in finding modalities that help you.

If there is no obvious reversible cause to your tinnitus—

First, remember that some tinnitus gets better or resolves with time. You could be one of those people. Also, research is ongoing, and some cure or treatment could be developed any time. Anyone affected with tinnitus should remain optimistic.

Otherwise, tinnitus treatment falls in several categories all aimed at reducing the perceived intensity of the tinnitus, and alleviating any adverse effects it might have on one's life.

Treatments for tinnitus

<u>Medications</u>

Unfortunately, there are no medications that treat or cure tinnitus itself, at least not at this time. Medications currently used for tinnitus include anti-anxiety agents such as alprazolam (Xanax), clonazepam (Klonopin), diazepam (Valium), and lorazepam (Ativan). Sleeping pills— eszopiclone (Lunesta) and zolpidem (Ambien)—are often prescribed for the sleep disorder often associated with severe tinnitus. Antidepressant medications, particularly some of the older tricyclic drugs, have also been found to be helpful to some tinnitus patient regardless of whether the patient has concurrent true depression.

While some people have claimed success with a variety of supplements and vitamins (including bioflavonoids and gingko), their positive effects haven't been confirmed in scientific studies.

How do I feel about medications for tinnitus? While I can't pretend to know your individual situation, I would suggest you be open to using medications if you need them, particularly when you first develop tinnitus. They can be life saving. They can alleviate some of the stress of tinnitus, and they can give you sleep that is so important. Also, if you have depression associated with your tinnitus, you should highly consider taking an anti-depressant agent.

That said—again, I don't know your situation—I would avoid taking medications for tinnitus on a regular basis if at all possible. Try to wean yourself off them, or only take them at times when they are absolutely necessary. My philosophy was that I didn't want to become dependent on taking medications for my tinnitus. All medications have some side effects. Many of the medications often used for tinnitus also cause withdrawal symptoms when stopped along with habituation (it takes more of the drug to have the same effect).

Each of us is different. Regardless of whether you use medications to help deal with your tinnitus, the principles and methods in this book can also aid you. Perhaps, for some, over a period of time less frequent use of medications will result.

Sound therapy

In its simplest form, sound therapy consists of the use of external sound (various white noise type sounds or music) to mask the sound of the tinnitus. The masking sound covers up or mixes with the tinnitus so that it is perceived as less intrusive—you can't hear the tinnitus as well or distinguish it as well.

Sound can either be supplied externally through any music or sound device or directly through the use of a specialized hearing aid.

Inexpensive noise generators are commonly available to provide external sound playing a whole gamut of different sounds and types of music. Similarly, computer and phone apps are available. Which sound is best? It is entirely subjective—whatever sound seems to blend in and cover your tinnitus best. Whatever you use, it is recommended that you use any masking sound at the lowest possible volume that gets the job done.

Many people find some sort of sound in the bedroom is particularly useful in aiding falling asleep.

Notched-music is a particular form of music therapy. In this, music or sounds with certain frequencies emphasized in a manner not perceptible to the listener are felt to aid in habituation.

Some hearing loss is often also present in many of those with tinnitus, and hearing aids can help mask tinnitus in two ways. First, the simple fact that hearing aids amplify surrounding sounds can help mask tinnitus. The tinnitus is simply not that loud anymore compared with normal sounds in the environment. Also, hearing aids are available with a specific masking component designed for tinnitus. An audiologist will determine the frequency and volume of your tinnitus, and the hearing aid will be programmed to play a constant low-level sound to help mask the tinnitus. In some, these hearing aid masking devices can also lead to some individuals becoming habituated to their tinnitus. Habituation refers to the brain reclassifying tinnitus as an unimportant sound that can be ignored. That is, the tinnitus no longer bothers some of these individuals as much, and they may be able to use the masking component less frequently.

Sound therapy is a complicated subject. There is much more detail on the topic of sound therapy and masking than I can present here, and I recommend you read and learn more about it. If you do use sound therapy, I advise you to strive to continue to learn and to maximize its effectiveness for your individual condition.

That said, my philosophy for myself—again, this is only my personal preference—was to try to limit and avoid masking techniques whenever I could. I didn't like the idea that I had to run and hide and try to cover up my tinnitus all the time. I realize this is touchy subject and each of us is different. I have used white noise next to my bed throughout the night, music and sounds while studying and background TV and other sounds in the house to try to cover the ringing in my ear at various times, but I wanted to avoid the path if at all possible of doing that *all the time*. I certainly make no judgment on what works for you.

<u>Avoidance of things that exacerbate tinnitus</u>

What can make tinnitus worse? Lots of things or nothing and it's different for everyone. Perhaps the most consistent thing is being in environments with loud noise. After exposure to loud noise, or even lower level background noise, for varying amounts of time, many people report their tinnitus becomes worse. Sometimes when it gets worse, it can be worse for days after exposure. As many people say, "I pay for it if I'm exposed to loud noises." Avoidance of loud noise, or simply any type noises that make their tinnitus worse, is necessary for many people, as are supplemental earplugs in certain situations.

Hyperacusis (mentioned previously and which often occurs in association with tinnitus) also makes it distinctly uncomfortable to be around loud noise.

Various food items or excessive amounts of them—notably caffeine, sugar, salt, alcohol—have also been associated with a worsening of tinnitus in some people. In some people, dehydration can play a role. Some people report allergies to various food items as worsening their tinnitus. Some people find that their tinnitus is affected by humidity or by barometric pressure. No consistent scientific evidence exists for any of these things, although this doesn't necessarily mean these things can't be true for some people. Later in this book, I will suggest you keep a log of your daily habits including what you eat, and attempt to discern any exacerbating factors for your tinnitus.

Behavioral therapies

It is notable that research shows little correlation with the loudness and pitch of a given person's tinnitus and the emotional and behavioral distress it causes. That is, one person can have very loud tinnitus (as documented by an audiologist) and not be bothered very much by it, while another person can have a quieter tinnitus, and have their life completely disrupted. We are all wired differently. Behavioral therapy for tinnitus generally involves helping a person *CBT* identify his or her response to tinnitus, and then attempts to reduce and correct negative responses that contribute to the disruption of life. The basic premise is that it isn't the sound of tinnitus itself that impairs our life, but rather our response to it. Cognitive Behavioral Therapy (CBT) and Tinnitus Retraining Therapy (TRT) are the most common forms of behavioral therapy. These and other behavioral therapies can either be done directly with a qualified therapist or through other means such as remotely over the Internet or via supplemental materials.

This book is most closely related to these therapies, and draws on many of the same principles. Any of the behavioral therapies would mesh well with the use of this book.

Other therapies

Basically, everything has been tried in an attempt to ablate tinnitus and diminish its effects on people's lives. This includes various types of surgeries, radiation therapy, any number of vitamin and herbal remedies, alternative medicine therapies such as acupuncture and homeopathy, relaxation techniques (yoga, meditation, mindfulness), hypnosis, and virtually any other therapy you can think of. There is always some person who got a beneficial result from any given therapy. Despite this, no clinical evidence exists to support consistent beneficial results at this time from any of these therapies.

The American Tinnitus Association (ATA) is a good starting place for an overview of tinnitus and various treatment modalities.

Which treatment modality should you use?

You may already be using some of these techniques. If not, research and find what works best for you. Any and all of the above treatment modalities may help you, and will not in any way diminish the effectiveness of the techniques in this book. Rather, they will work in concert with this book.

So Where Are We Now?

This book presupposes that you have had a thorough evaluation for your tinnitus and that there are no reversible causes. Again, don't shortchange yourself in getting a thorough workup. This book also assumes that you may or may not use any of the above treatment modalities along with this book. Again, they all work in concert with the strategies in this book.

But first, in the next chapter, let's look a little more closely at how tinnitus often *does* affect our lives, and not shortchange the fact that it is a real and sobering dilemma to most of us.

Chapter Three

It's A Big Deal

If someone develops tinnitus and they tell you it's no big deal and they can just handle it, I say they are full of it. It doesn't happen that way. Tinnitus *is* a big deal. I'm not talking about some mild buzzing in your ear, but I'm talking about a full-on loud, high-pitched, all-encompassing shrieking in one or both ears that makes it next to impossible to do anything. EEEEEEEEEE! And it is there all day and all night and back again when you wake up in the morning. If someone says *that* isn't disturbing—earth-shaking disturbing—they must live in a different world than you or I. Or they are lying.

Let's think about it for a moment. If you are someone who just developed tinnitus, it is normal to be alarmed. In fact, something would be wrong with you if you didn't react that way.

All our lives, we are accustomed to hearing things and responding to them. We are accustomed to being able to turn off noisy items or get away from them. We may be stuck in a noisy environment but we know eventually the noise will subside or we will be able to leave. We know we have control. We may have to accept noise for a period of time, but we know eventually it will end.

Also, noises—particularly loud constant ones—are often

signals that we need to do something. Think of fire alarms or sirens. They are a warning that something is wrong and we need to react. We are wired that way. So tinnitus *is* something unique and out of the ordinary; it doesn't follow our standard rules.

✓ It is an important first step to accept the fact that it's not your fault the way you may respond to tinnitus. There is nothing wrong with you. The way you are responding is normal. It's natural.

And no matter how or when tinnitus started for you, it never starts at a good time. There is no good time to get tinnitus.

And It Does Change Your Life

For most people with severe tinnitus, it does change their lives. Big time. In a major way. If you have severe tinnitus, you could probably separate your life into two segments: the time before tinnitus and the time after tinnitus.

The loss of true silence, which is so precious to most of us, can feel devastating. It *is* sad, heartbreakingly sad for many of us, the fact that we can no longer just sit and be in silence, that we no longer can *not* hear anything, and that it might stay that way for the rest of our lives. We know we have to learn somehow to accept that, but, nonetheless, it is hard.

If our tinnitus is severe enough, it may cause us to have to change our job, hobbies or lifestyle. It may affect our relationship with our spouse or friends. It may certainly affect our home situation and how we sleep or have to sleep.

The hyperacusis (increased sensitivity to noise) that is often associated with tinnitus may cause us to curtail social gatherings or going to certain environments that we used to enjoy or limit aspects of our job or occupation.

And it can certainly make us depressed and discouraged.

You Don't Look Sick

Another one of the unique aspects of having tinnitus is that we don't look sick. We don't limp or shuffle. We don't gasp for air or have any obvious deformity. We all look like normal people. Standing in a grocery line, working at a desk, driving a car—no one would be able to tell that there may be a loud, unrelenting noise in our ears. No one else can hear it. There is no evidence. Despite our ringing, we often suffer in silence. This is one of the peculiarities of tinnitus.

There Is a Time to Feel Sad, Angry, and Depressed.

When we first get tinnitus, it is natural to feel overwhelmed. If you are like most people, in one form or another, I believe we all go through something akin to the Elisabeth Kubler-Ross's famous five stages of death. The stages are denial, anger, bargaining, depression, and acceptance. You may go through them fast or slow, in order or out of order, in greater or lesser degrees, but I believe all sufferers of tinnitus go through them in one form or another. Indeed, some part of you does die when you get bad tinnitus. Things change. Your world isn't the same as it was before.

But going through these various stages is a healthy normal process. We have to go through these stages to some degree before we are fully ready to work on solving our tinnitus. So while this book will help anyone with tinnitus no matter where they are in the process, I believe it is important to allow yourself to go through these stages, and this process unfortunately often means hurting and feeling bad. This is the part of the process of coming to grips with your tinnitus.

During denial, we say things like the following to ourselves (or others): This can't be happening. I can't imagine something this bad, this loud, this disturbing not stopping. This can't or shouldn't be happening to me. Why is this happening to me? I want to go to bed and wake up and it not be there. I want to go back to my old self. Yesterday, one week ago I was perfectly normal, now everything is seemingly irrevocably changed forever.

The second stage—again, we may not go through them in order—is anger. We say such things as: This isn't fair Why me? I hate this. God, I hate this. I don't deserve this. I wish this would happen to someone else. Or our anger can spill out to other people: I hate life. I hate people. I hate everything. If I'm feeling this bad, I will make sure everyone else feels bad too. Why did this happen now? I'm too young to get this? I'm too old—I don't need this now. Why can't any of the doctors help me!

The third bargaining stage includes some sort of deal with a Higher Power. We say something like, "Look, God, if this goes away, I will live a better life. I will be a more compassionate and caring person. Okay?" Looking for a cure—not in a rational manner, but in a desperate, frantic manner—may be included in the bargaining stage. We may try or do virtually anything. For many of us in this stage, we, unfortunately, find nothing really helps.

Then, in stage four, many of us become depressed, deeply depressed. *We truly are stuck with this.* That thought is so very frightening and overwhelming that we often have no reference with which to handle it. Imagine living like this for the rest of our life, we ask ourselves. And the answer is, I can't, or at least at this time, I don't see it as a possibility. Tinnitus can suck the life out of one's life. The sky is no longer beautiful. Things we used to love and care about can suddenly seem lifeless, and all the stuff people involve themselves in become vapid and meaningless.

Or the depression can be a subtle, low-level depression. It can be more like a bitter resignation to one's fate as it were.

But let me say this right now. If you have tinnitus and you feel severely depressed and suicidal, *do whatever it takes to stay alive.* And I mean whatever it takes. I don't want you dying over this stupid tinnitus. It is not worth it. Go to an emergency room, call a suicide hotline, stay with friends, take meds, get help from your doctor, see a therapist, do anything and everything. And do it right now. This is not the time to be brave or noble. Do whatever it takes to get help. True depression is a tricky rascal. Something is tricking your brain into feeling something that is not true. Don't fall for it. Don't accept it. Get help somehow some way—but get help now. It may sound glib for someone to say it will get better but it will and it's true. No matter how bad you think it is now, ✓ you can and will get better. You will be able to handle it. You will have times again when you aren't bothered by tinnitus at all. Hang in there. Know—trust me—that if you do things to get through these tough times, you will survive and you will be glad you did.

With all these stages, there is grieving. Some people cry—I certainly did—for what is lost. We cry, we grieve for what is changed because of the pain, because of the anger, because God doesn't answer, because of the depression. We don't feel good. Let yourself grieve, be angry, and maybe depressed. Let yourself hurt.

Going through these stages hopefully allows us to reach the final stage: Acceptance. We may have this forever. We may not. But this is the hand we are dealt. Acceptance is what makes a situation, while perhaps not preferable, at least okay.

Some people may not ever quite reach this stage, or may cycle back through previous stages or even make one of them their home. They get stuck or frozen in one of the earlier stages. For example, some people might get stuck in the anger stage. They become angry over their tinnitus, and they *stay* angry. They become bitter people or have hidden passive-aggressive, under-the-surface anger, which spills out into all other aspects of their lives: family, friends, work. You don't want to do that.

Or another person might become stuck in the depression stage. They tell themselves at some deep level that because they have tinnitus they can, should, or have to be depressed. You don't want and don't need to do that either.

Ideally, we all want to reach the acceptance stage: I have this. I wish I didn't, but I do. Now I'm ready to do all I can to deal with it.

Identity Ailment

Over the years working in the emergency room, I saw many people who identified with their diseases or disabilities. Their disease or disability became *who they were.* And while I am in no way belittling anyone's suffering, over time I recognized that those who thought of their problem simply as something they had or that was bothering them did better than those who identified with it. Those who identified themselves with their ailment allowed the problem to control and define their lives, most often in debilitating ways. Their identification with the ailment (this is who I am—a person with such-and-such disease) compounded and made worse the effects of their original problem.

We all know people who identify with their ailments. For example, someone with chronic back pain will preface everything they say with the fact that they have chronic back pain, or someone with fibromyalgia (a sometimes debilitating disease) will continually point why they can or cannot do something because of their fibromyalgia. Or another person might have been in a bad car accident in 2002, and their whole life since that time remains in reference to that event. Again, I'm not making light of these problems. But rather than being Bob or Sue or Kevin, these people become, in their own minds, a-person-with-chronic-back-pain-who-will-never-get-better, or a-person-with-fibromyalgia, or a-person-who-is-the-way-he-is-because-of-a-car-accident-in-2002.

I refer to this as having an identity ailment. By this, I mean identifying with your ailment to such an extent that it becomes a huge part of who you are. There are many people out there who do identify with their tinnitus. Their tinnitus is and remains a big part of their life, of who they are and of what they think they are capable of doing. For example, aside from truly offering to share and help others, who would want to hang out on a tinnitus forum? Who wants to live the remainder of their life talking to people about a stupid ringing (that no one else can hear) in their ears no matter how severe?

For some—not all—of the people particularly on the Internet, there is even a perverse sense of glee in having something. "I *am someone* because I have tinnitus." It almost becomes a badge of honor. They have an identity in a group. Or they play the game of "my tinnitus is worse than yours and I've had it longer."

Hanging out either online or in person with other so-called "tinnitus sufferers" can be a drag. It can bring you down. The problem is that when we see or read about other people responding to tinnitus in a certain way, that sends a strong subconscious message to ourselves that that's how we need to respond. It's almost as if we are children and all the adults in the room are acting a certain way, and hence, we pick up on and decide and assume that's the way we should act too. We think, "That's the way I should feel and be too."

While there is value in knowing that others have what you have and perhaps picking up some tips or techniques in dealing with tinnitus, we don't want to buy into any negative gestalt about having and living with tinnitus.

Some people may also justifiably (or not) blame their tinnitus on the fault of someone else in the past, a dangerous work environment, or perhaps even on mismanagement by a health professional. Yes, it *is* unfair and perhaps terribly wrong that this happened to you. People were bad. Mistakes were made. But somehow you have to find a way to let it go eventually. When the time is right, *you have to let it go.* Because "All the time you spend tryin to get back what's been took from you there's more goin out the door,"—Cormac McCarthy, *No Country For Old Men.* The price you end up paying is your life going out the door. You can't afford to let that happen because of tinnitus.

So don't allow your tinnitus to develop into an identity ailment, and put aside whatever may have caused your individual tinnitus. Do this *for yourself.* We can have tinnitus, but it is *not* who we are, and the fact that we have tinnitus does *not* define our life or what we are capable of.

Some people can even want to keep their tinnitus or to keep letting other people (and their own self) knowing that it is bothering them.

Secondary Gain

Part of the process of this book is to weed out and destroy ⲦⲂⲦ
any negative ways of looking at things that might limit our
handling of this tinnitus thing. Secondary gain refers to when
there is actually some advantage, some benefit, to keeping or
persisting in a seemingly detrimental behavior.

So let me ask you a question: Why might someone *not* want
their tinnitus to go away, or why might someone *not* want to
be able to handle it?

Stupid question, you might say, everybody wants it not to
affect him or her.

Well, when I first started having my tinnitus, I got a lot of
sympathy from my wife, and it was justified. I felt terrible
and I did need help. Her support and reassurance did make
a difference through those hard times. But I could see how
that could become a habit, my saying "poor me" and she
consoling me. I didn't want to live like that, but some people
might. We have to be on the look out for becoming addicted,
as it were, to any sympathy others might give us because of
our tinnitus.

Or maybe tinnitus could become an excuse for not doing
everything you need or want to do. We'll talk more about
this later. "This ringing is so bad, I can't possibly _____
(fill in the blank)." Maybe you *allow* your tinnitus to keep you
from looking for a job, finding a good relationship, being a
good partner or parent, or simply being the happy person
you were designed to be.

Tinnitus could also keep us from growing, from taking that
next step in our life. It can be the perfect excuse; only we can
hear it, so nobody can ever doubt how much it bothers us.

Some people—myself included—just like to have things to

worry about. Tinnitus can fill that need.

So become aware of using your tinnitus in some way unfairly to your advantage. If you really can't do something because of the ringing, that's fine. But if any way, you are milking tinnitus for your advantage, don't do it. Stop it.

Summary

After reading this chapter, you should be aware that tinnitus is or can be a big deal, and have some awareness of the stages we all go through in adjusting to it. You also should be aware of the pitfalls of an identity ailment, and secondary gain. Now we're ready to move forward.

Chapter Four

How This Book Works

This chapter is the time when you as reader and I as author huddle together and outline our strategy.

It's like our tinnitus is over there and out of range and can't hear or see what we're planning. We nod and agree with each other. I explain some things to you. You ask a few questions. Then we shake hands or high five each other and get to work with the rest of the book.

How Do We Define Success?

How do we define success in dealing with our tinnitus? We want one of three things or some combination of them. The first possible definition of success would be for our tinnitus, for whatever reason, to go away completely, and we are never bothered by it again. For some people, that is a real possibility. Or, similarly, that it physically diminishes in intensity enough (again, for whatever reason) that it no longer bothers us.

The next way we might define success is that despite having tinnitus, despite hearing the ringing in our ears, we are not emotionally wrapped up in it. It does not negatively affect us or distort our lives. We want to change the way we feel and react when and if we do notice our tinnitus.

Finally, the third possibility is that we become habituated to our tinnitus to such an extent that we don't notice it's there. It's still technically there, ringing away, but we don't focus on it. We functionally don't hear it. This is akin to a tree falling in a forest and no one being there to hear it fall. If tinnitus exists and we don't listen to it, for all practical purposes, it doesn't exist.

While I can't predict whether your tinnitus goes away or diminishes in intensity, through the use of this book, and perhaps other modalities, you should certainly expect to decrease both your emotional response to tinnitus, and to functionally hear it less and less.

It's Not A Battle

With regard tinnitus, I don't like the idea of battle. I don't like the idea of fighting tinnitus, or even of trying to conquer it. I don't believe an adversarial attitude is helpful, and hence, I avoid words like battling tinnitus. Rather, I like Sun Tzu's *The Art of War* idea of defeating an enemy without even fighting it. Or I'd also go a step further. We aren't going to defeat it. We are going to adapt to it in such a way that it has little or no effect on us. If all goes well, you may be able to say most or all of the time, "I don't really know whether it is there or not, and I don't really care either."

Have you heard of the martial art called Aikido? One of the tenets of this discipline is that you don't head-on confront a force with opposing force. An example would be when an assailant attacks you, you step aside and allow and redirect the assailant's forward momentum to move him out of your way.

That is something akin of what we want to do with our tinnitus. We want to gently yet resolutely redirect the effect tinnitus has on us into a new positive direction to our benefit.

We *do* want to fight that we will not allow tinnitus to adversely affect our lives, but we want to do in a way where we accept that it is there.

This might sound confusing to you, but as we go along, you'll get the idea.

A basic tenet of this book is that the way you are mentally responding to tinnitus isn't working as well as it could, or could use at least some improvement—or you wouldn't be reading this book. So we have to accept from the start that we have to do things differently. We have to both think and physically respond differently to our tinnitus than the way we may have in the past.

Another way of thinking about it is that we want to rewire our brains—sounds scary, doesn't it?—to be on our side. For example, you might say we want to remove some wires from where they are attached and reattach them to different locations. Some wires we just want to leave dangling with no place to go. We want to think differently about tinnitus.

Certainly, many people do end up accommodating to tinnitus on their own and over time, but we want to accelerate that process. We want to super-charge it, while at the same time consciously incorporating strong mental habits into our psyches.

The Three Basic Principles of this Book

Principle Number One

Handling tinnitus is in great part a mental game. No matter what other adjunctive therapies we may use, we want our minds to be on our side. We want to represent things to our advantage. We want to use techniques based on the ways our minds work to both diminish our hearing of tinnitus and to diminish the effect tinnitus has on our lives.

Regardless of whether you have just developed tinnitus or have had it for a long time, you need to be open to the fact that the way you think—through no conscious fault of your own—can contribute to your feeling bad with tinnitus. Think of this as an opportunity. We want to sever any connections we can that contribute to our feeling bad. We want to maximize our minds' role in handling tinnitus.

Again, regardless of the severity of your tinnitus, this can only help. This will move you in a positive direction.

Principle Number Two

You have to believe things can get better. No matter what your individual situation, things can get better. We can handle this. You can handle this. If you feel you are beyond hope, if you feel you can't take it anymore, if you feel you want to give up—you aren't, you can, and don't!

And if you've had tinnitus for a long time, this book can be an opportunity to reevaluate the ways you are thinking about tinnitus and dealing with it.

Things can change. For some, whatever is causing your tinnitus can stop. You don't know everything. Are you God? Something caused it to start; something can cause it to end. There is always hope. There are many people who had tinnitus, and it went away. You may very well be one of those people. And even if you think you are not, you still may be. Miracles *do* happen. Cures *are* found. Even right now, doctors and scientists are working feverishly for a cure for tinnitus. They might find something—today. Things do change.

The next moment, the next day, the next week, the next

month can change everything. Month, you might say, I can't survive a month more of this. I know how that feels too. Let me say this for anyone who is suffering right now. I remember one morning when I felt so hopeless and depressed I could hardly get out of bed. Another day of just trying to survive this wretched noise in my head, only to survive enough to eventually struggle to go to sleep and then wake up and have it start all over again! I almost did feel like killing myself. But then a few hours later for some reason—I don't know why— the ringing lifted a little. I could see the sky and people and everything was magically reasonably back to normal, to the way it used to be. And I thought, "Jeez, I was so bad off an hour again, and now I feel back to normal. How could I have thought that way?" Later, the ringing came back in full force but it made me think that there is always hope. It made me think things can change.

And even if for whatever reason, you don't believe that your tinnitus may get better on its own, there are ways and techniques to markedly diminish big-time both noticing that you have tinnitus at all, and to diminish or get rid of any negative effects it has on your life. You can get to the point where you forget about your tinnitus.

You have the power and the resources inside you to do this. Even if you may not feel right now that you have the power and the resources to do this, you still do. This can get better. We can make this get better.

You're bigger and more powerful than you think.

Principle Number Three

Little things we do to change the way we represent tinnitus to ourselves lead to big changes over time. Little changes we make in the way we deal with tinnitus add up and make a difference in tinnitus' overall effect on our lives.

I've been listening to a song lately. Part of the chorus is, "It's the little things you do." It's the same thing with our tinnitus. We all want some big glorious cure-all for our tinnitus, such that it instantly never bothers us ever again, but it doesn't usually work that way. It's the little things we do.

We can and will do big things to diminish tinnitus' effect on us, but at the same time it's the little things we do over and over that begin to have a cumulative effect on controlling it. Principle number three says that anytime we do any thing, *any little thing*, even once, that helps to diminish the effect tinnitus has on our life, we need to recognize the importance of that and how it leads to our long-term success. Any small step we take is worthwhile. Any time you use one of the methods in this book, it is worthwhile. We do one thing, it helps some. We do another thing; it helps in a different way. There is a synergistic effect. We can't always predict how things are working beneath the surface. But the methods in this book can and will work to move you in a positive direction.

One of the characteristics of tinnitus is that we generally don't notice all the times *we aren't* bothered by the tinnitus. Little changes, little steps, lead to these times we aren't bothered becoming more frequent and lasting longer. We generally might not notice this right away. Only after a period of time, we might say, "Hmm, you know I haven't thought of or been bothered by tinnitus for an extended period of time."

This book has a number of techniques. You can't always be sure which methods will work best for you. Even if you think you know, you might be wrong. That's why I suggest using them all. Not to sound too mysterious, but some of them work beneath the surface, beyond your conscious awareness. And again, one mental technique accelerates the effect of another mental technique. Be open. Let things work. The idea is that we keep hammering away from every direction, knowing that after a certain point, all these methods will reach a critical mass and things will tip in our favor.

Or to put it another way: It's a numbers game. The more times and ways you consistently do small things using different mental and physical techniques, the faster you will diminish the effect tinnitus has on your life, the quicker your overall success. It's the little things we do.

Openness

Think of a storeroom jam-packed with boxes and various other items. Everything is so tightly packed in the room you can barely move around in the room. Fitting anything else in the room would be hard.

That's the way it can be with regards our tinnitus. We can quickly become so jam-packed with opinions on how tinnitus is and has to be that there is no room for other possibilities or solutions. Many of our opinions may be valid, but often there is little or no room for other ways of looking at things.

So first we have to make some room for other possible ways of thinking about our tinnitus and for other solutions we may not have thought of. In fact, I'm going to move you from the jam-packed storeroom to a huge, high-ceiling, empty warehouse. You can bring all your boxes and stuff—in fact, I want you to bring all your stuff with you—and put it somewhere in the vast warehouse. Put it in a corner or spread it out. You immediately notice it doesn't take up too much space.

That's the way I want us to be. I want us to have lots of room around us to move and stretch and try out new ideas.

Another analogy for this openness is when you are learning a new sport or activity, how you need to be open and also give your body and mind some room to figure things out. For optimal results, you can't go into the learning process having a preconceived idea of how things should be, how you should hit a tennis ball, for example. While learning, while being taught, you have to make room for the process being slightly different than how you might have thought. And you have to give your body time and space to integrate what you're being presented with and to figure things out in its own way.

It's the same thing with the techniques in this book. Be open.

It Has To Seem Weird or Different

You know the old maxim: If you keep doing the same thing, you keep getting the same result. By definition, we want what we do to be different. Some of the things in this book may seem weird, outrageously stupid, or just plain silly. "That can't work," you might say. Some of the methods in this book may even seem beneath you. But our minds are often simple and child-like in that way they work. Cerebral arguments rarely work particularly in dealing with something like tinnitus.

Which again leads us to—

✓ But You Have to Do Your Part

This getting better, this learning-how-to-handle-tinnitus, is a participatory sport. You have to get involved yourself. You have to get down on the ground, get your hands dirty a little and get involved. Put on your work clothes. Be open and have a sense of curiosity and playfulness.

The more you fully participate, the greater the results. You have to get individually involved because the way your tinnitus affects you is unique to you. I don't know exactly how

you think, so your job is in part to customize many of the
methods in this book to fit yourself. Your specific thoughts
and ways of looking at things are part of what we are dealing
with here.

Read this book and do the exercises when you are alert. Do
any exercises that are prescribed with full participation. Give
yourself the gift of allowing this stuff to work.

Many of the exercises in this book will require you to write
things down. Get a notebook. Don't write on scraps of paper.
Take it seriously. The things you write and the observations
you make can and will change your life.

One other caveat before we get started—

Maybe Don't Share Too Much of What You Are Doing With Others

What? We are always told to share things with our family
members, friends, and spouses. That's a healthy thing, isn't
it? Well, not always.

See, for some of those with tinnitus when you are starting off
doing the things in this book, you are a like a tender sprout
just pushing its way through the soil up into the sunlight. A
plant like that is easily destroyed by any number of things. Too
much or too little water can cause it not to thrive. Any small
environmental change can jeopardize its growing. Whereas
a larger plant may easily bounce back is pushed on or even
stepped on, a small plant doesn't yet have the resilience to
survive much. It's just getting started on its path.

It's the same with you and this process. Some may be a bit
frayed around the edges (to say the least) from this whole
tinnitus experience. You are vulnerable. Your grasp on dealing
with tinnitus, albeit, even surviving it some days can be quite

tenuous. When something begins to help, when something has the possibility of helping you, the last thing you want is for someone to make some aberrant remark or comment, no matter how well intentioned, that may jeopardize your fragile recovery. "Oh, you're trying to think positive—that's good," they might say for example. But that's not really what this is about, and other people's glib pronouncements on what you are doing or should be doing are probably not helpful at this stage.

They—other people—don't really know what you are going through. They aren't experiencing what you are experiencing. They can get some glimmer of it from your description, but they don't *feel* what it is really like. So I suggest you at least consider keeping most of what you do in this book private, for yourself at least for now.

Remember principle number three—it's the little things we do. Even just by reading this and starting this process, you are sending the first of many strong messages to yourself (and to your tinnitus) that it isn't going to run rampant. You are in charge.

Chapter Five

Our Bodies and Minds Are Adaptable

You know it really is amazing how adaptable the body is. It is amazing how we are able to habituate to stuff, to get used to it. It is as if our body tells us, "Okay, initially that was novel or dangerous or different, but now I see it's not a problem. I can disregard it."

People work in factories with constant, loud noise. At first, when they just start working there, the noise is overwhelming but over a period of time, they don't notice it anymore. Their minds tune it out. People live next to busy roads, near train tracks, and airports. I remember visiting my Uncle Al and Aunt Dorothy who lived next to the airport in Milwaukee. Planes were taking off and landing all the time—Al and Dorothy couldn't care less and didn't even notice. Or have you ever been in a noisy bar and had a particularly interesting conversation with someone. All the loud music, the clanking of glasses, the loud talking and laughter—it was all tuned out.

Some people work around noxious smells, bad odors, stuff that stinks real bad all day. Again, at first, I'm sure it's a shock, but after a period of time they become used to it and, again, don't even notice it. After a long enough time they might even ask you, "What smell?"

Have you ever walked through swampy water, let's say up to your thighs? At first, it is creepy. The water is cold and bits of grass and vegetation continuously rub past your legs. Ick! But if you stay in the water eventually you don't notice it anymore. Again, your brain tunes it out.

People can work in dangerous situations. For better or worse, after awhile they often don't notice the danger anymore. It is as if our brains are lazy and say, "I can't keep up the effort of being upset about this if it's not going to change."

People eat weird, exotic foods. If we ate them, we might find them unpleasant. But after a time, people get used to eating almost anything. Heck, what first tasted terrible, sometimes over time becomes our favorite food. Strange, huh?

Have you ever seen a wound heal? If all is going well, usually it begins to heal around the edges. New skin begins to form around the edges. The wound doesn't really go away, but rather it slowly gets covered up and replaced with new skin starting at the sides and moving toward the middle. And it all doesn't happen all at once. It takes time but not too much time.

Or sometimes when a certain part of our body is used a lot, we grow callouses on that part. We become hardened in that area so that we aren't as sensitive in that spot, and things just don't bother us as much.

Chapter Six

Why?

Why do you have to handle this tinnitus thing in your life?

Because it's a nuisance and it's driving me crazy. That's a good reason . . . but not good enough. See, our reason for doing something is like the under-the-surface engine powering the whole machinery of accomplishing something—in this case, limiting and diminishing the effect tinnitus has on our lives.

So I want to play a game with you. Play along with me on this. I want you to pretend you are standing in front of someone who can magically control the effect tinnitus has on your life, but first, you have to convince him or her that you sincerely want it to go away or for its effect to markedly diminish in your life. Now this person sees lots of people every day who want their tinnitus to diminish. Some people come in and say something like, "Yeah, it's really bad and bothers me, and if you could make it go down, I'd like it." But our magical being isn't swayed by that type lukewarm argument. He or she is looking for people who really with their whole heart and soul want it to diminish. Magical power isn't something to be used lightly or on a mere whim.

So what would you say? Go ahead—you're up. What words would you say or use? How would you convince this being that you want the effect tinnitus has on your life to diminish?

Write down exactly what you'd say in your notebook. What are your reasons? Are your words forceful enough? Do you think the person would be convinced? Try to dig down and get to the real reasons why you absolutely, positively 100% must diminish the effect this has on your life. You have to convince our imaginary person (and yourself) that you really want to handle this.

Maybe you can remember some time in your life when you wanted to do something—no, not just wanted it, but needed it, decided you were going to do it, refused to accept 'no' for an answer. *It was going to happen.* There was no question of you giving up or not getting what you wanted. You focused on it with unbending intent; you were going to get it. Perhaps as a parent, you wanted to provide something for your child, and you worked harder, saved money, did whatever it took to make it a reality. Or maybe you hit some sort of low in your life, and said "I'm not going to take this anymore for myself. I am simply no longer willing to accept this for myself." That's the kind of intensity we want in handling this tinnitus thing.

Or maybe some people depend on you now. They need you. You just aren't willing to let them down by your becoming absorbed with your tinnitus. You can't afford it. They are more important to you than yourself. Or maybe you just want to be an example to others.

Hopefully, when you write down your reasons, you use phrases like—I must do this. I have to do this. I refuse to accept anything less. My life is too precious. I refuse to have this mess up my life. I simply will not allow it.

The magical being is listening intently and leaning forward in his or her chair.

Ask yourself a few more questions: Who are you anyway with regards to getting things done? Who do you want to be with regards to getting things done? What are you willing to accept for yourself? What are your standards for yourself? Is that who you are—someone who will be controlled by tinnitus? You wouldn't be reading this book if you were.

No matter what your life is like, we've all had moments when we've lifted ourselves to our full height and power. That's the person I want you to remember and be. It is not consistent with that person—with who you really are—to act defeated or discouraged with regards tinnitus.

Back to the magical being who seems swayed by your argument. Now he or she asks, "But what are *you* willing to do?" It's as if you've passed the first part of the interview. Now if you can only answer this second part equally forcefully.

The magical being knows tinnitus can be challenging to deal with. He or she doesn't expect superhuman abilities, but just consistent, unwavering intent and action.

How would you answer? For your part, what would you say you are willing to do to handle this?

Here's part of what I come up with for myself: I will do whatever it takes. I will not be defeated. I will not accept not handling this. I will handle this. I don't have time for anything less. If I ever feel discouraged by this, I will pick myself up as soon as I am able, and continue relentlessly at finding ways and reinforcing ways not to have this adversely affect my life. I will keep looking for new techniques and practicing those that work.

Are your statements similar to mine? Write down what you are willing to do.

The other side of motivation, the deeper darker side, is: What is the cost if we don't handle this?

The magical being (who is actually your own self) waves his or her cape, and you become shrouded in dim light . . . and you see what your future will or could be like if you let tinnitus take control of your life. What if you *don't handle this?*

For myself, I see myself spending inordinate amounts of time thinking about tinnitus, listening to the noise of it, and feeling depressed and discouraged. I see myself over time become more and more discouraged and upset. I see myself not getting along with people the way I used to because "I have tinnitus." I see my home and family relationships suffering. I see myself doing poorly at work—after all, I have this burden that others don't have that I must shoulder. I see myself hating myself inside because of all this, and hating life. I see myself not doing all the things I want or need to do. I see my identity becoming wrapped up in the fact that I have tinnitus. I see myself not being the person I could have been and not living my life to the fullest. Perhaps I even start drinking or using drugs too much, and this spirals me further down. Not a pretty picture—not who I want to be.

What will your life be like if you don't handle this tinnitus thing? Might your future be something similar to mine to some degree? Look into the shrouded light that magical being created and see your future if you don't handle this.

Write down all the negative repercussions if you don't get your tinnitus under control. What will your life be like? How will you feel about yourself? Do you want to be that person? How much of your life in the future do you want to be absorbed by worrying about tinnitus?

Hopefully, you are as depressed as I was thinking about that future. The magical being waves his or her cape again, and suddenly we are in sunlight under a bright blue sky. Now let's continue.

Chapter Seven

What Do You Believe?

If we want to get rid of tinnitus or minimize its effect on our life, it can be hard or impossible if under the surface we have beliefs that essentially sabotage this from occurring. It would be like trying to build a house with a faulty foundation. Even if we construct exceptional walls and roof, our house just won't be solid.

Or it is as if on the surface we do things to diminish the effect tinnitus has on our life, while under the surface we have core beliefs that say, "This can't really work," or "This can only help so much." Part of us wants to go one way, but part of us is preventing us from fully going in that direction. We want to clear that up. We want our underlying beliefs to be our allies in our dealing with tinnitus. We want our beliefs to be on our side.

Beliefs, in general, are our deep-down convictions about how things are, about what is or is not possible, and about how hard or easy it is to accomplish something. They could include such ideas as "People are inherently good," "We can only control things so much," or "It's impossible for me to change that." Our beliefs are the linchpins in our psyches that control (and help create) our reality. And in a sense, we all go around carrying our sacks of beliefs representing who we are and what we think we can and cannot do. Many of our beliefs we share with other people. They have the same beliefs that we have, while some of our beliefs are unique and personal.

The thing about our beliefs (yours, mine, ours) is that we think that they represent the way things *really* are. I do. You do. We all do.

We may have gotten some of these beliefs growing up from those around us. We may have created some of these beliefs ourselves when we went through trying times in our lives. In essence, they are ways we chose to represent things, and, hence, they control our reality.

The problem with our beliefs is that some may not accurately reflect reality or what is possible. We may develop beliefs that are not conducive to us solving our problems. Our beliefs can keep us stuck. If you drive a car one time and then decide it's too dangerous or you are not coordinated enough, then that might be a silly belief to have. That belief about driving may not be a *useful* belief to have. It won't allow us figuratively (and literally) to go in the direction we want to go.

So—and here's the key thing—*we want to have beliefs that are in our favor. If we don't have them, we want to make them.*

I'm going to repeat that in a slightly different way—*if we don't have beliefs that are in our favor, we want to create them and make them part of ourselves.*

But you might immediately argue, "That's not true or fair. You can't just make up beliefs!" But I would argue back that we actually do it all the time, make up ways of looking at the world based on the flimsiest of evidence or experience, and keep and preserve them for years. We have to *decide* to create positive beliefs for ourselves.

Do you remember the first *Matrix* movie where Morpheus explains to Neo that what is holding him back is simply what Neo believes he can or cannot do? It's the same with our beliefs. Many of them hold us back from what truly is possible. Or we may think certain things have to hurt or mess up our lives.

And—you probably know where I am going with this—we also have beliefs about tinnitus, the possibility of it going away, and about our ability to control and diminish its effect on us. We have, or have developed, all sorts of beliefs about tinnitus.

So first we want to become aware of what beliefs we do have about tinnitus and our being able to control or diminish its effect on our lives. Then we want to replace any non-constructive, feeling-bad beliefs with more powerful beliefs that will aid us in handling this tinnitus thing.

So what are some of the beliefs you have about tinnitus and about being able to handle it and live your life to the fullest? Write down all your beliefs, both positive and negative, about the way you think about tinnitus.

If you are or were like me, your beliefs might be something like these.

This is a bad thing, and I am unlikely to get better.
One can only do so much to deal with this.
This is going to destroy my life in a big way.
No one can really help me.
When I hear the ringing in my ear, I become upset and depressed.
There is nothing I can really do to help.
People who deal with this are stronger than I am.
This is essentially the end of my life. It will never be the same again.
I'll be stuck wearing a hearing aid and listening to white noise all the time.

Yes, I may survive this, but my life will be messed up.
I won't be able to do many of the things I like doing ever again.
I will never feel happy.
There truly is no real help.

Did you write down your beliefs? If someone had beliefs like mine (and perhaps yours), how likely or unlikely do you think it would be for that person to learn to deal with their tinnitus?

If a person, for example, has a belief that says, "I'm stuck with this, and to a certain extent I'm going to have to fight this the rest of my life," is there a chance that would become their reality? Or would that at least contribute to their reality, and perhaps keep them from making maximal progress in dealing with tinnitus?

And now for a few minutes—similar to the previous section on motivation—I want you to think what will be the cost if you keep having those negative beliefs about tinnitus. What price will you pay long-term? How will it affect your life—will it make your life better or worse if you hold onto those ways of thinking about tinnitus? Will those negative beliefs make it easier or harder to feel better?

Wouldn't it be a shame if you had some lousy beliefs or ways of thinking and they contributed to your staying stuck in tinnitus for years or for longer than you had to? That would be a real tragedy.

What I want you to do now is to take each one of your negative beliefs about tinnitus and put some holes in them. I want you to explain on your paper why each one may not be true, or may not be true all the time. Write down several reasons for each of your negative beliefs individually why they may not be true. This may be hard to do. You might not see right now why they might not be true. That's why they are our beliefs. We believe them! But I need you to find some reasons why they might not be true. Create some doubt over why they might not be true.

For example, if I believe because I have tinnitus, I *have to* feel bad, I would write down some arguments of why that might not be true: there are people out there who have tinnitus and don't feel bad; just because I hear a noise, I don't have to feel bad about it necessarily; people work in environments where there is loud noise all the time, and they don't feel bad. I've just created some doubt in my cherished belief.

Or another example, if I believe I can never get better from tinnitus, I would write down such things as follows: people get better from things all the time; things *do* go away; no one has all the answers; if I don't notice my tinnitus, it is effectively gone away.

Here's another example. Perhaps I tell myself that because of tinnitus, I can't live or do all I would have otherwise. I could counter that belief by writing such things like this: lots of people with problems go on to do *even greater* things than they would have otherwise; maybe because of this I could become a better person; maybe having this will allow me to grow in other ways; maybe I could use this as a reason to live my life to the fullest.

What I want you to do is just to create doubt. Demonstrate that your old negative beliefs may not be the only way to think of things. Another more graphic analogy for what we are doing is bashing the legs off the belief system table that holds up our way of thinking about tinnitus.

What if we all had beliefs that were on our side in dealing with tinnitus? Given a choice, why would we not want to have beliefs that *help* us in dealing with tinnitus?

Now I want you to go back to your negative disempowering beliefs and alongside each one write a new belief that would be advantageous to your getting better, or looking at tinnitus in a more positive, constructive way. Write beliefs of how you would like to look at things. Write beliefs about the optimal ways you might view things.

To repeat—I don't want your new beliefs to be necessarily 'fair', and they don't need to seem entirely rational right now. That's why they are new beliefs. They will probably feel different. I want your new beliefs to be in your favor, to your advantage.

If you have a little trouble with this, that's okay. We're trying to take our minds and wrench them into a new position. It might feel weird. And if you've had your tinnitus for a long time, it might be harder to come up with new beliefs, let alone convince yourself of them in the section that follows. Changing a long-held belief, or even coming up with a new possibility, would be akin to a large cargo ship turning while at sea. It takes time.

Here's another tip. Remember our new beliefs do not need to be 100% valid and reasonable. Sometimes the more bizarre and nonlinear a new belief is, the more it actually appeals to us and sticks in our brains. For example, if I say, "Because I have tinnitus, I can allow myself to feel happy more often," it doesn't make complete sense, does it? But it can work.

Finally, write down what would be the advantage if you had those new beliefs. Would it be possible that you could handle this tinnitus thing more adeptly? Would there be even one situation in which instead of looking at tinnitus in a disadvantageous way, you'd see it in a better way? Might one of those new beliefs pop into your head at a time when you might feel overwhelmed by tinnitus, and steer you out of it.

Even once? Could that make a difference in your life? If that feeling of looking at it in a better way occurred numerous times over days and weeks, would you be in a different, better place than you might be otherwise?

First, here is one key belief we all need to have—the Master Belief. Here is it—the key belief we need to incorporate into our lives: I can have ringing in my ears, but I don't need to suffer or feel bad because of it.

Read that again. Read that a few times. Write it down in big bold letters. That is a main point of this book. That is what this book is about. That is what we are trying to do with many of these methods. We are breaking the link, cutting the connection, between noticing the ringing in our ears and feeling bad.

Or to say the same thing in another way—

I can have tinnitus but I don't need to feel bad, bothered, upset, angry, mad, depressed, or discouraged. I can feel those things if I want . . . but I don't need to.

Or to expand on that—

My tinnitus can be loud and high-pitched and last all day, but I don't need to feel bad because of it.

Do you remember that unequal symbol from when you took math in school—the equal sign with a slash through it? Write the word "ringing" in your notebook, then write the unequal symbol, and then write the word "upset." Ringing does not equal being upset. Ringing does not have to equal being upset.

Ringing in the ears is a physical sensation. Our response to it is emotional. Some wise person said, "Pain is physical. Suffering is mental and optional." Hearing or noticing our tus is physical, but how we respond to it is up to us. At making this distinction on a practical day-to-day level may seem difficult or even impossible (or even make you mad that someone would even suggest it). We certainly can't just say, "Okay, it won't bother me anymore," close this book and go home. Rather, there is a knack to doing it. But for starters, let's always keep that belief in the back of our heads: We can hear our tinnitus, but we don't need to be upset by it.

Along with this, we have to recognize that at some level *we make ourselves* feel bad about tinnitus. Again, we don't like to admit it. I certainly didn't like to admit it, but I eventually had to acknowledge that I was, on some level, doing much of this to myself. I was in some way, even though it was initially beyond my control, causing myself to feel terrible. Not totally, not entirely perhaps—but I had something to do with it. It is an important initial step to begin to acknowledge this.

Listen right now for the ringing in your ears. Find it and listen to it. Now think to yourself, "I can hear this, but I don't need to be upset by this." Try to feel what I am talking about for just for a few seconds—I can hear this, but I don't need to be upset by this.

So what follows are some beliefs that I have come up with for myself. I've come up with lots of new beliefs. You can use them as a template to develop your own new beliefs. They fall in several categories. Many times I say the same thing in slightly different ways. Again, remember, the value of a belief is its ability to empower us to go in the direction that we want to go. Read over my beliefs slowly, and when you are done maybe add to or modify your own new beliefs.

The first group of beliefs has to do with the master belief, separating the hearing of ringing in our ears with feeling bad.

Not Having to be Upset by Tinnitus

I can hear the ringing in my ears, but I don't need to feel upset by it.

I can hear it, but I don't need to be upset, bothered, angry, discouraged, or depressed because of it.

I can hear it loud or high-pitched, but I don't need to be worried, scared, mad, or overwhelmed.

I don't have to feel bad because of this.

My tinnitus can be loud and persistent, but it doesn't have to bother me.

Just because I happen to hear ringing in my ears does not mean I have to be disturbed by it.

I can hear ringing in my ears and not be disturbed.

I accept that I have this, but at the same time, I don't need to be bothered by it.

There is an attitude available to me right now where I don't need to be upset or bothered by this. I can find that place.

I can hear it, but I am not upset anymore.

I don't need to fight and struggle with this. I can if I want, but I don't need to.

I don't need to be fearful about this. I can relax and rest despite any sound that I hear.

I don't need to be upset or bothered by this anymore.

Having tinnitus may not be optional, but feeling upset because of it is optional.

I *don't have to* feel glum and morose because of this. I can if I want to, but I don't have to.

Next are a series of positive beliefs about our ability to handle tinnitus and the possibility of the tinnitus going away or not bothering us.

We Can Handle This

I have the resources to handle this.

I trust that I can handle this so that it doesn't bother me anymore.

I have faith I can handle this.

I am handling this.

If I hear it, that means I'm handling it.

I give room for things to happen in a positive way.

Even if I hear the ringing and even if it upsets me sometimes, everything I am doing is still working.

I can handle this. I have handled difficult challenges before, and I can handle this too.

I am open to different ways of handling this.

I am flexible in my approach to handling this.

I am open to this resolving.

Each day in some way I am getting better at handling this.

I am gentle and loving to myself for having this.

I am open to things getting better at any time. My tinnitus may go away completely, diminish in intensity, or can completely stop bothering me in any way.

This can effortlessly get better.

I am open to this getting better in a surprising way, when I least expect it, and faster than I can imagine.

Next are a few beliefs that reinforce our taking any action to handle this.

Taking Action to Make This Better

Anytime I do any small thing, even once, to diminish the effect of this on me, I take a giant stride forward in resolving it forever.

Little changes in the way I think about this can have big effects.

Little actions I take can have big effects in diminishing the effect this has on my life.

When things are worse, and I do something to handle this, my actions have even greater results.

I support and reinforce myself for any step, no matter how small, that I take in looking at this differently or disrupting my old way of thinking.

I will keep a log and do all I can to discover anything that makes my tinnitus worse, and take action to avoid or prevent those things if possible.

I may not always recognize how much progress I've made in handling this. Each day despite any setbacks in some way I am getting better at handling this.

I give my body and mind time to integrate this so that it doesn't bother me.

I have set in motion a process for this to resolve and to diminish any effect it has on me. Even when I am not aware of it, things are working under the surface to accomplish this.

If I do one thing one time to not become overwhelmed by this, that is great, and I support myself in taking any small steps in handling this.

Each day in every way I am moving closer to not being bothered by this.

The more I enjoy the day, the more this goes away.

Each day the effect this ringing has on me is getting less and less.

Anytime I interrupt the pattern of being upset by this, that has a massive effect on this not bothering me.

If I am briefly bothered and upset, it doesn't matter. I am still moving in a positive direction to resolve this.

There is a process I have put into motion where this doesn't have to bother me anymore.

The fourth group of beliefs has to do with why we simply will not accept or allow tinnitus to control our lives in any way.

Tinnitus Will Not Control My Life

I refuse to allow ringing in my ears to diminish my life in any way. I will simply not accept that for myself.

There are things I want and need to do in my life. I will not let this stop me or slow me down in any way.

I allow myself to be undisturbed by why I got this or why this happened.

I simply will not accept being bothered by this. I don't have time.

The louder my tinnitus is, the more empowered I become.

The next group of beliefs has to do with how having tinnitus could allow us to grow and become better people. What meaning could we give to our tinnitus that is positive?

Tinnitus can change our lives. For some people, they *do* have to give up certain activities because of it. While I encourage you not to do this prematurely, it is a fact for some of us. But while we may be forced to change certain aspects of our lives, tinnitus doesn't have to change who we are inside. And it can allow us to grow and expand in other dimensions that we may not have been able to otherwise.

I talked to a man who had to give up playing the piano because of tinnitus and its associated hyperacusis (sensitivity to sound). He ended up finding another outlet for his creativity and emotional expression. Matisse, the famous French painter, became disabled later in life. Unable to paint, he still created, producing his famous cut-outs, which some claim are his best works. "Une seconde vie," (a second life) he called it.

If we are in some way thwarted in the way we do something by our tinnitus, perhaps we can find a different and even better way of doing it. Again, tinnitus may alter your life, but it doesn't have to alter who you are and the expression of your unique gifts.

Some people may need to change their occupation or give up hobbies or activities they used to love because of tinnitus. Some relationships may not be exactly the same before and after the development of severe tinnitus. Some of us may have to accept that, while at the same time not allowing it to diminish us as who we are. We can become bitter, or we can see it as an opportunity to grow in new, unexplored ways.

Tinnitus could be the thing that allows you to grow in a new, different way in your life. It could make you into a more compassionate, caring person. It could allow you to see the suffering that is all around that you may not have been aware of before. It may spur you to take action to help people in different ways (as it did for me). It could force you to reevaluate your life, and decide what is truly important to you. Tinnitus could serve as a wake-up call.

Whether you are religious or not, I believe there is some truth in the statement that when God closes one door, another door is opened. We need to find the door that has been opened.

Here are some beliefs related to how we can grow and become better people *because* of tinnitus—

Growth As a Person Because of Tinnitus

In some way I can grow and become a better person because of this.

This can be a wake-up call for me. Because of this, I can do even more than I would have otherwise.

Because of this, I can allow myself to live my life to the fullest.

Because of this, I allow myself to do more, to feel more happiness, to be more vibrant and alive.

I am open to somehow finding the good in this and growing as a person because of this.

I accept that somehow there is a positive unfolding in my life with this occurring.

Because of this, I can allow myself to be happy all the time.

Because of this, I can decide not to worry about things as much.

Because of this, I make it a point to do one thing, in particular, each day where I help others and am a positive influence.

If you want you could even decide that your tinnitus represents secret messages coming only to you from outer space or something. It's probably not a good idea to share that belief with other people, however . . .

Or that you're lucky to have tinnitus. Why? I don't know why. Make up a reason—any reason.

The final group of beliefs has to do with what I would call the spiritual side of things. Obviously, you have your own spiritual or religious beliefs. If specific religious principles are part of who you are, by all means, incorporate those views into your beliefs about dealing with tinnitus.

The Spiritual Side of Things

I am grateful every day for all that I do have.

I send loving healing thoughts to my body and myself. There is a power to love that automatically allows the best outcome to occur.

Somehow in some way, I am guided and protected.

My intention is aligned with the Universe and is working to resolve this and allow me not to be affected by this.

Do any of my beliefs resonate with you? Now, as suggested previously, go back and refine and improve on your new beliefs. Your new beliefs should use words that fit with who you are, words that you like and that have meaning for you. The exact wording of my beliefs probably won't be exactly right for you, just as yours may not be exactly right for me. Another way of saying this is that our new beliefs have to feel congruent with who we are or, in this case, who we want to be. Our words need to perfectly mesh with the optimal way we want to view the situation. When we read one of our beliefs, we don't want to any glitch inside that says "That's not quite right for me." Remember, these are the beliefs we want to have; these are the beliefs we *need* to have. Take some time in doing this. Write out your new empowering beliefs with authority and conviction. Write them out for what they are— the new ways you have decided to believe about tinnitus.

Now that we have our new beliefs, it is not enough to just let them sit there in our notebooks. We have to make them real for ourselves. We have to repeat them over time. We have to reinforce them in ourselves. We have to make them become real for ourselves until they become who we are and what we believe.

What? You're going to want me to repeat my beliefs over and over with some sort of religious fervor, and that's going to change my tinnitus magically? Well—sort of and yes.

By repeating and affirming our beliefs, we help create that reality. We are telling ourselves that this is how we are committed to things being. We are creating a positive future with regards tinnitus. We are being resolute in how we want to—now from this day forward—view our tinnitus.

Does repeating our beliefs with authority and conviction work? Of course, it does. If we repeat something to ourselves with firm conviction, it *does* become our reality. Athletes and other successful people do it all the time.

The key point in making our new beliefs real for ourselves is when we read them or repeat them aloud or internally, we want to *feel* them. We want to connect with feeling that new way emotionally. We want to feel the essence of the belief inside ourselves even for a few seconds. We want to feel it as true. This often means taking a slight pause, perhaps closing our eyes, and feeling what it feels like to have this new belief. We want to make that emotional connection when we repeat our beliefs each and every time.

So if I read my new belief that says, "I am open to somehow finding the good in this," I want actually to stop for a few seconds and feel that. I want to feel, "Yes, there is a way, and I will find good in this."

When is a good time to read or repeat your new beliefs? The morning is an ideal time to do it, to start the day setting the stage for how you are going to respond to and think about your tinnitus. How many beliefs do you need to repeat? As many as you want, but over time you may find that some resonate more with you than others. Depending on where you are with your tinnitus, some of your new beliefs might feel more necessary at a given time. Some, over a period of time, may not feel quite right to you, or you may not need them anymore, and you can put them to the side.

As you go on through this book and in the time ahead, develop new beliefs that continue to move you in a positive direction. After a time, however, you may not need to read your beliefs as much. When you think of that aspect of tinnitus (how you feel about it, what it means to you, etc.), you will automatically think of your positive belief. It will become who you are in relation with tinnitus.

Your beliefs are the underpinnings for all that follows. Make them positive and to your benefit, and reinforce them until they become part of who you are.

Chapter Eight

Can I Ask You A Question?

How often have we had someone say that to us? Well, that's exactly what I'm going to do in this chapter. I'm going to ask some you some questions, give you some of my answers to them, and then encourage you to ask and answer your own questions.

Are there people out there who have tinnitus as bad as you do, and who have learned to handle it so that it doesn't bother them at all?

When I asked myself this question, I had to answer yes. I'm sure there are people out there. But maybe they have stronger minds than I do, or maybe they simply have more resilience than I have. But then I had to think—maybe some of them are just like me. What did they do and how did they do it? I asked myself another question.

Who are some people that I could think of who could have tinnitus and not be bothered by it?

When I asked myself this question, I immediately thought of Spencer West. I had just read about this incredible human being who at an early age had the lower half of his body amputated from his pelvis down. He has gone on to do fantastic things, both achieving personal goals and helping countless people on several continents, all the time dragging himself around with just his hands. I thought to myself, "If that guy got tinnitus, it wouldn't bother him in the least. It wouldn't stop him at all." There are lots of people like Spencer who have disabilities greater than I could imagine who somehow live happy, productive lives.

The next group of people I thought of was some of our military. Many of them come back from combat with traumatic injuries such as terrible burns, amputated limbs, and brain injuries. And many of these great warriors refuse to lose a step in getting on with their lives. They know that others of their kin gave the ultimate sacrifice and that they are lucky to be alive. Because of this, they refuse to indulge in their injuries. For many of them, this resilience is part of their training and their pride of both who they are as individuals and of their units. Many of these men and women would not let something like tinnitus slow them down or affect them in the least.

The next group I came up with when I thought about this question is people, particularly parents, who have to take care of their children. When a child is sick, or when a single parent is trying to raise a child despite overwhelming odds, the parent simply doesn't have the luxury of worrying about his or her own problems. One simply has to put one's own problems aside. There are bigger, more important things to do. Or if by having this tinnitus somehow I could save the life of someone I love, I would do it in a heartbeat.

Finally, I thought some people might just get tired of giving tinnitus emotional energy. They get tired and even bored with it. It's simply too much trouble.

This led to my asking myself another question: Under what circumstances would I see my tinnitus as a good thing. At first, I thought "under no circumstances!" But then I began to think. If I was paralyzed, but then somehow recovered and was only left with this tinnitus—well, I'd be the happiest man in the world. I would think this is "nothing" compared to what I did have.

What if I was in a wretched prison serving a life sentence. Would I trade getting out of the prison for having this tinnitus? Of course, and would I be bothered by this tinnitus? No, I don't think it would bother me at all.

Finally, I thought in answer to my question, there are simply some people who are so busy living, who have so much to do and that they want to do, that they would absolutely refuse to be slowed down by something like tinnitus. They are just too busy and happy living to allow themselves to be affected by it.

Write down your answers to the questions:

Are there people out there who have tinnitus as bad as I do and it doesn't bother them? Who are they?

Why doesn't it bother them?

How do they think about it differently than the way I am thinking about it?

What would make me think my tinnitus was a good thing?

How could I apply some of the qualities of these people to my own tinnitus situation?

Is there some part of the way those people think that resonates with me?

How can I—even in some small way—think the way they think?

Questions bring up possibilities. They begin to make us think that there are other ways to relate to our tinnitus. Part of the strategy of this book is to put as many chinks in the armor of your tinnitus so that you can't quite think about it in the same way as you were before. Questions cause that to happen.

Here are some more questions.

I believe we all have an intuitive sense of what is the best way for us as individuals to handle something. I believe we all *secretly* know what would work for us. So let me ask you—

What is the best way for you to handle this tinnitus in your life?

What would *you have to do* to handle this?

What steps and techniques would you have to take?

Spend some time thinking and write down your answers.

Some people might say, "Well, I don't know—hey, that's why I'm reading this book!" But let me go a step further to try to root out some of what you might already know about what works for you, and ask another question.

Even though you don't know what would help make you deal with this, if you did have to make your best guess, what would that be?

How about this—imagine all the super-smart people at all the best high tech companies (Google, Apple, etc.) gathered together in an auditorium. The leader comes out and says, "Okay, here's your assignment," and they all momentarily lower their phones. "Your job is to come up with the most fun, imaginative way to make ringing in the ear *not* bother a person. What might be some of the ways they might come up with to handle this?

Write down some of the novel ways they might come up with dealing with this.

Another question—

When you have handled challenges like this before in your life, what did you do? How did you do it? What worked for you?

What resources did you use?

If you were designing a plan for someone you truly love to deal with this, what might you prescribe?

Sometimes the military talks about outflanking an enemy instead of attacking them from the front. How might you outflank the negative effects tinnitus has on you?

Again, write down your answers. Play around with these ideas in your head.

What if you did just keep slowly, methodically applying the techniques in this book, would that make a difference over time in your tinnitus?

Is there any idea so far in this book that particularly appeals to you?

Here's an interesting question.

Why do you feel that you have to react to tinnitus in the way that you do?

Maybe at some deep level, we *do* feel the tinnitus represents a threat to us. Maybe some deep part of ourselves is telling us over and over this is bad and we need to react this way to it for our survival.

How might that not be true?

Maybe it is not really a threat. Maybe our brains can interpret it that way, but maybe it really isn't a threat when we think about it logically. In fact, maybe some of our thinking of it as a threat is what keeps it being a threat. Maybe it was okay to think of it as a threat in the past, but we don't need to now.

Here's a question—how long does it have to take you to control the effect tinnitus has on our life? How long does it have to take to handle this?

Weeks, months, years? Or maybe your answer is you'll never totally handle it. That's okay too. Just become aware of how you are thinking.

How could you go all out in handling this? What would your plan and strategy be? What would you do if you could do anything? What keeps you from doing that? How might you get around any perceived obstacles?

How hard is this to handle? On a 1-10 scale, how hard do you rate it? What if it actually is easier than that? What if it actually 3 levels easier than you think?

We touched on this in the chapter on beliefs but how could you think about tinnitus so that when you noticed it, you not only didn't feel bad but instead you felt strong and empowered? How would you have to think about your tinnitus to feel that way?

Would it be possible for someone to hear their tinnitus and notice it and feel more vibrant and more alive? Could their tinnitus trigger them into living their life to the fullest?

Or we could take it a step further—

We touched on this before, but is there some way because of having this that you could become a better person than you would have been otherwise?

Maybe you could become more compassionate. Maybe you

could understand other people's suffering more than you did before. Maybe you could help more people. Or maybe on a personal level, you could realize that life truly is short and this could spur you on to do greater things, and to live your life to the fullest. Maybe.

Finally—

If you did handle this tinnitus thing, how would that make you feel about yourself?

Play with all these questions in your head for a little while and write down your answers. Also, I suggest you go back after a day, a few days or a week and answer these questions again, and see what you can discover.

Chapter Nine

The Power of Words

Words have power, not only the words we say to others but also the words and phrases we say to ourselves inside our own heads. Words create our reality. Words create pictures in our brains, and our perception of reality conforms to those pictures.

If we tell ourselves something is "driving us crazy," it will tend to drive us crazy. If we tell ourselves something is "mildly annoying," we are more likely to feel—well—mildly annoyed.

So we want to start becoming aware of the words we are using to describe our tinnitus and its effect on us. Sure, when we first develop tinnitus, we might tend to say it's terrible or horrible, and use other similarly emotionally-charged words to describe our reaction to it. Because it is! But after we decide to do all we can to control our response to tinnitus, we have to become conscious of our language, and it helps to purposely use words and phrases that convey diminished emotional intensity. We need to consciously change any words or phrases that we use that are overly negative or that perpetuate negative emotional states into ones that don't make us feel as bad. Again, we are not only talking about the words and phrases we might use when talking to others but those that we use inside our own heads, our self-talk.

One way we can do this is by simply picking a word that conveys a milder version of our original (often overly dramatic) emotional state. Angry becomes annoyed. Overwhelmed becomes inconvenienced. Terrible becomes trying. We want to make the language we use concerning our ringing and its effect on us less emotionally intense. Another thing we can do is to purposely use understatement and humor in our language when we talk or think about tinnitus to decrease the impact it has on us. The British in particular often have a knack for this, this art of combining understatement with humor in a way to diminish an effect something has on us. I even imagine there must have been some Brit during the bombing of London during World War II who referred to it as a bit of a nuisance. That's what we want to start to do with our tinnitus.

Let's look at the word tinnitus itself. Kind of an ugly word, and if you are like me, it certainly has come to have a negative connotation particularly when I first began to have my ringing and was reading all the invariably-depressing forums and medical information on the Internet. It is such a somber and serious-sounding word no matter which of the two variations of pronunciation you chose to use.

For starters, you might want to choose a different word to refer to your tinnitus for yourself. Maybe call it a "hum" or "a faint buzz" or just call it a "little sound." Even the word "noise" can be a bit disturbing; we don't want to call it a noise. How about calling it a "background sound?"

I know some of you out there might immediately say that your tinnitus is neither faint nor small, that my new words are not accurate, and that this won't make a difference. But I ask you to at least play along with me and try this. Remember, little things do make a difference.

The reason this is important is because we don't want to give the ringing in our ears more energy than we have to, and part of the way we do this is through the words we use. This is yet another way we can start, through the words we use, putting chinks in tinnitus' armor.

So right now think of several different words you might use to refer to your tinnitus. Here are some other examples—that background buzzing I sometimes hear, a faint humming, a mild background sound, a gentle, hard-to-notice murmur.

Be imaginative. Come up with three of four different word or word combinations for your ringing. Make sure that the words you pick make it smaller and less significant than it might have been otherwise. Consider starting using those words now and for the rest of this book when referring to your tinnitus for yourself. (However, for rest of the book I will continue to use the word tinnitus for simplicity).

What about phrases we might commonly say to ourselves and others when talking about our tinnitus? Is tinnitus "destroying our life?" Would it be better to say, "It's a tad irksome sometimes?" Is it better to say, "This is keeping me from doing anything!" or "It can be a bit of a nuisance once in a while, but doesn't stop me?" Again, even if you don't believe it right now, just start to purposely use less-intense words and phrases to describe tinnitus' effect on your life.

What are some phrases you currently use to describe your experience of tinnitus? Write them down. Look at them carefully. Might your phrases be in some small way contributing to keeping you stuck? Now write down some better less-intense alternatives.

Sometimes our repetition of certain phrases become so set in our minds that they become what Tony Robbins, the motivational speaker, refers to as incantations. Think about tribesmen dancing around a fire rhythmically chanting the same phrase over and over. Similarly, we can repeat certain phrases over and over in our heads usually with a certain cadence and tone of voice that it is as if we are trying to call forth some mumbo-jumbo spirit. Or to put a spell on *ourselves*. We essentially summon and perpetuate a certain feeling in ourselves.

Here, for example, are some of my old incantations. Here are some of the phrases I used to repeat over and over in my head.

"I can't take this any more. I wish someone would help me."
"I can't survive like this."
"This is terrible."
"This will never get better."
"I hate this."
"My life is ruined."
"What am I going to do?"

When I was saying these things to myself, I would invariably say them in my head in a certain tone of voice with a certain hopelessness and helplessness. Saying these things would make me feel miserable. And they weren't helping me to get better.

Are there any incantations that you repeat to yourself when your tinnitus feels overwhelming? Again, they need not be as dramatic as mine. Just the fact that you say them over and over is what makes them significant. Write them down. And when you repeat your incantations, what tone of voice do you use in your head? Bring them out into the open. Often by simply realizing what we are saying to ourselves—by bringing them out into the light of day as it were—they lose some of their effect on us.

Hopefully, you will find this curious in an interesting sort of way. Our minds and the way we use them certainly are strange things. And while you are certainly entitled to keep repeating anything you want, you may become aware that these phrases—like all incantations—certainly may also be contributing to keeping us stuck.

What if you tried not to repeat some of these phrases to yourself, or tried to make up different better ones? Even if you only did that—changed what you said to yourself—once or twice a day, could it make a difference in your reaction to tinnitus? How about if it made you chuckle to yourself when you caught yourself and used your new, improved phrase? Might that help even a little? Maybe it could even cause you to laugh a bit at your own response to tinnitus?

If you want to change your incantations, try to use the part of your original negative incantation so that when you start to say the bad one to yourself, it's easy for the new improved positive incantation to insert itself. Rhyming helps a lot.

It's almost as if you sidetrack or divert the incantation in mid-stride.

Here are some examples using some of my original phrases and others.

"I can't take this anymore" becomes "I can't fake this anymore."
"I can't survive like this" becomes "I can thrive because of this."
"This is terrible" becomes "This is actually quite bearable."
"This will never get better" becomes "There is a distinct possibility that this will improve immensely."
"My life is ruined" becomes "At times this is a tad disconcerting."
"What am I going to do?" becomes "What am I going to do? Perhaps go to the zoo."

"It's so loud" becomes "I'm so proud."
"I'm sad" becomes "I'm glad I'm handling this."

You get the idea. So, first, what you want to do is come up with some alternative phrases for yourself. Then when you catch yourself repeating and old incantation, you want to repeat your new phrase instead, or if you want you can repeat both your old phrase and your new phrase together.

This does two things. It allows us to catch ourselves when we are stuck using our incantations in a relative, unconscious manner. By becoming aware of what we are doing (saying to ourselves), we become less emotionally caught up in the negative emotion, or, hopefully, not at all. We also start disrupting our negative patterns.

Or to put the point of this chapter in the simplest terms: We don't want to be saying stupid things to others and to ourselves that help keep us stuck in feeling bad about tinnitus. How's that?

Changing the words and phrases we use is one step in minimizing tinnitus' effect on us.

Chapter Ten

Don't Give It Energy

Have you ever seen one of those science fiction movies where an alien entity threatens a group of space travelers, and despite all their best efforts to fight it, the alien entity only grows in strength and power? The more they fight the alien, the more it grows in size and power until it threatens the space travelers' existence. Finally, someone realizes that it is the fighting with the entity, the giving of attention to the entity, which gives it power. The entity *feeds* on attention, and that is what allows it to grow in size.

So our intrepid space travelers stop focusing on the alien entity. They purposely stop giving it attention. They recognize it but they stop fighting it, and the entity shrinks, diminishing in power and strength until it finally becomes either insignificant or disappears in a poof of space dust.

That is what we are trying to do with our tinnitus. Recognize it is there but do all we can *not* to give it energy. Every time we give it undue energy or attention, we allow it to grow and gain more control over us.

We aren't running from our tinnitus. We aren't afraid of our tinnitus. But rather, we simply want to smoothly, efficiently deal with it in ways that curtail its influence over us.

So one of the first things we can do to help handle our

tinnitus is to deal with it in a matter-of-fact way. We simply do whatever we feel is necessary at a given time, but we don't make a big deal of it.

For example, I may be working on something and notice my tinnitus. Without making a big deal of it, I might put on some background music while I am working. No big deal. No excessive thinking about it. Just do it and keep on working.

Or maybe (I'll talk more about sleeping later) I might have trouble falling asleep because of the tinnitus. Rather than becoming overly frustrated and struggling for a long period of time, I might just take a sleeping pill. Again, no big deal, no struggle. No giving any additional energy or focus on the tinnitus than is necessary.

Or maybe you use some of the other adjunctive treatments for tinnitus. Quickly, efficiently, practically use or do whatever is necessary. Don't make a big deal out of it. No internal whining, worrying, complaining, getting depressed—just do what you need to do the best you can.

Or maybe I'm at a location where the noise is exacerbating my tinnitus. Again, in a matter-of-fact manner, I might use earplugs to help, leave the location, or if I am unable to, simply accept the fact.

Here's yet another example. Perhaps you are in a situation where your tinnitus is bothering you for whatever reason. If you can, why not just get up and do something else. Distract yourself. It's an absolutely fair strategy to purposely do something else when you feel you are prone to focusing on your tinnitus too much. Why linger with your tinnitus if you don't have to. No need to. No reason to. Why hang around listening to it. You can listen to it if you want . . . but it's actually kind of boring. Why not just put yourself in another situation where your tinnitus may not seem so intrusive?

And, again, do it in such as way such that you remain cool and collected. Don't hurry. Don't become frantic. You want to maintain an air that you are the calmest, most serene person in the world. Even if you are a tad distraught, you want to *pretend* to yourself that you are not. Don't give your tinnitus that unnecessary emotional energy.

One elderly gentleman I spoke to who had tinnitus for many long years gave this advice: "Ignore it." If you can, use his ultimate method of not giving tinnitus energy—simply ignore it. Then the gentleman added, "And if you can't ignore it, go do something else like watch a football game." All good advice.

It is as if we are trying to become Zen masters in the way we deal with our tinnitus. We don't make a big deal in our heads about what's going on or what we are doing. We simply take the action that we think is appropriate at the time, and then leave it and move on.

This creates non-attachment to our tinnitus. It is almost as if it is not us. We deal with it the way we might deal with a problem at work; we simply handle it or chose our best option in handling it at any given time. If water is leaking, we turn off the faucet. If it's too bright outside, we put on our sunglasses. We avoid becoming overly belabored in dealing with tinnitus. We intentionally refuse to allow it to garner our emotional attention.

The more we do this—not making a big deal out of our tinnitus—the easier it becomes to do this and the more we gain control over tinnitus. Every time we deal with our tinnitus in a practical, simple, matter-of-fact way, not giving it excessive energy, the more its power and control over us diminishes.

So our first rule for this chapter is—do whatever you deem

best to handle your tinnitus at any given time in a practical, matter-of-fact manner. Don't give your tinnitus unnecessary attention, focus, or energy. Don't add any emotional overlay to what you are doing—just do it.

The second part of this is that maybe sometimes our tinnitus, for whatever reason, does seem to overwhelm us. That's okay. Let it. Accept it. Maybe sometimes you try to use some of the adjunctive methods to treat your tinnitus or the techniques in this book, and they *don't* work. Maybe sometimes you just can't handle your tinnitus in an emotionless, matter-of-fact manner. You *do* become depressed or discouraged for a period of time.

We are emotional beings; that is part of who we are. If you become upset, let it be.

Again, try not to make a big deal of it. Feel depressed or discouraged and then as soon as you are able, move on and don't look back. Let the episode of feeling distraught fade away. Don't dwell on it. Don't worry about it. Forget it. And do this every time you might feel depressed or discouraged— as soon as you are able, move on and don't look back. "Okay, I felt bad today. Big deal. Now I am going to move on."

Making a big deal out of the times we don't feel good is giving the alien entity energy in another way. We don't want to do that. As soon as we gain any amount of strength and focus again, we go back to our usual ways of dealing with our ringing.

So our second rule of this chapter is—don't make a big deal over the times you feel bad with your tinnitus. Move on and don't look back.

Similarly, don't make a big deal about whether something you do for your tinnitus works perfectly or doesn't in a particular instance. For example, in the next chapter, I will talk about interrupting the pattern of feeling bad or focusing on your tinnitus. Sometimes, particularly when you are just starting out, it's difficult to interrupt your patterns. Don't make a big deal out it. Don't get discouraged. Just keep trying. What we are after in the long run is persistence. Just keep doing things to the best of your ability. That is enough.

So we have yet another rule—don't make a big deal in your mind if a given technique works perfectly in a particular instance or not. Consistent effort is what matters the most.

Finally, it is easy for some of us to become overly obsessed with tinnitus. We read books (this one is okay!), read stuff on the Internet, and do other things that make tinnitus too much of a focus in our life. Recognize that this is another way we might be giving tinnitus more energy than we should.

So our final rule for this chapter is a hard one (more of an art form): to find the balance between doing all you can for your tinnitus while at the same time not becoming fixated on it in a way such that you give it uncalled-for energy.

Chapter Eleven

Interrupt It!

Some of you reading this may be suffering right now, so I'm going to give you a seemingly simple technique that will work at least some of the time (if not much of the time) in dealing with a negative response to tinnitus. In later chapters, we are going to expand on this but right now here is something you can do.

It's simple. Every time you catch yourself feeling bad about tinnitus or focusing on it too much, interrupt it.

First, I want you to recognize, regardless of how bad your tinnitus may be, that there are times—many times—when you are upset by your tinnitus, and something interrupts the way you are feeling and you are forced to forget about your tinnitus for a period of time. You may be dwelling on your tinnitus, and then, let's say, you get an important phone call. You completely forget about your tinnitus while you are talking on the phone. And you do this forgetting-about-your-tinnitus very fast, in a split second. This fact provides the basis for what follows.

But before I go into more detail, let's play another little game—

What if I told you that every time you became upset by your tinnitus, you had to do a certain, very specific prescribed ritual? You had to act out a precise, detailed set of instructions. What would happen?

So here's the ritual I am prescribing for you to do whenever— that is *any time every time*—you feel overcome by your tinnitus.

Immediately stand up.
Walk counterclockwise in a small circle four times.
Reverse direction and walk clockwise three times.
Stop.
Face north—you might want to carry a compass with you at all times.
Repeat the phrase, "I shall not be bothered by tinnitus" twice.
Then stamp your left foot three times while exhaling sharply.
Then sit back down.

If after doing this and sitting back down, you again feel your tinnitus bothering you, guess what? That's right—you have to get back up and repeat the whole ritual immediately. This time, however, you stamp your right foot three times instead of your left foot. You alternate sides each side you do the ritual!

I'm being a little tongue in cheek here obviously, but the point is it would quickly become such a nuisance to do such a stupid ritual, that we would either pretend we aren't being bothered by our tinnitus or simply truly stop being bothered by it. The hassle of having to do the ritual would outweigh allowing ourselves to feel overwhelmed by our tinnitus.

The point is that there *are* things we can do to interrupt our tinnitus in such a way that we can and would avoid focusing on it. If we make it awkward enough for ourselves to keep doing a behavior, we will change it or stop it. And if we interrupt a pattern enough times, it will be hard for it to run anymore.

Simply put, the more you interrupt the pattern of feeling bad, both the amount of time per incident that you feel bad *and* the number of times you feel bad will begin to decrease.

Again, remember, we only tend to focus on all the times we are distracted by our tinnitus, not on all the times that we forget about it, even for a few minutes. Each time we interrupt one of our negative tinnitus patterns and keep it from starting and running its whole length and go back to what we were doing, then that is one more segment of time we *weren't* distracted by our tinnitus. Those begin to add up.

It works like this—

Notice your tinnitus and start to feel bad.
Interrupt the pattern.
Go back to what you were doing.
Time passes.
Notice your tinnitus and start to feel bad.
Interrupt the pattern.
Still noticing your tinnitus and feeling bad.
Interrupt the pattern again (and again if necessary).
Go back to what you were doing.

After awhile, you only have to give yourself a sense that you're going to interrupt the pattern and your brain stops focusing on the tinnitus as much. Our brains begin to say, "What's the use of doing this if it's just going to be interrupted again."

How do we interrupt a habit or pattern of feeling bad over tinnitus?

Any way we can.

Instead of using the long ritual above (you could if you want), we can basically do anything surprising and out of sequence that keeps us from going down our negative tinnitus response pattern. Specifically, we purposely do anything or say anything that momentarily distracts ourselves. We move differently. We say something aloud. We focus on a distant object. We stamp our feet. We do an irrelevant mental calculation. We try to remember a distant memory. Generally, the more bizarre and out of context the thing(s) we do, the better this technique works. Doing several bizarre, out-of-context things in a row works even better. Also, you don't have to do the same thing every time. You don't need to be consistent or methodical in your plan. Be unpredictable to . . . yourself. Surprise yourself in the different ways you interrupt negative tinnitus patterns.

Here's how it might work for me. For example, while studying I'd start to listen for my tinnitus and then start to feel bad. Immediately, I'd purposely say a funny word or make a funny face. I would move my eyes from side to side. I'd stare out the window and try to identify an individual leaf on a tree. I'd stamp my feet, or move my arms vigorously. I'd point to the ceiling. Or I'd try to remember the capital of South Dakota. I would quickly immediately do anything to distract myself, to interrupt the pattern of focusing on and feeling bad about my tinnitus.

Then I'd start studying again. If I began to hear or focus on the tinnitus again, I'd immediately do more out-of-context, bizarre actions to interrupt that pattern. Again, do I do the same thing every time? No. I make up anything on the spur of the moment. Again, it doesn't matter what you do—just do any quick little thing(s) to interrupt yourself from listening to the tinnitus and feeling bad.

At first doing this takes some effort, but over time it becomes easier and more automatic to interrupt the negative patterns. At first, you may have to do this interrupting lots of times.

It may seem like you are doing it all day. But—trust me—as you keep doing it, you will need to do it less and less. The spaces during which you are not being bothered by tinnitus will grow and expand.

As mentioned above, what began to happen by doing this is that many times after just doing this brief interrupting technique, I'd go back to studying or whatever else I was doing and forget about my tinnitus for a period of time. The amount of time I was disturbed by tinnitus became less, and, over time, the number of times I was being distracted by the tinnitus became fewer.

Was I initially able to do this technique 100% of the time and make myself stop being distracted by the tinnitus? No. But it began to work most of the time.

This is not a cerebral technique. We don't want to think about doing this; we want to actually do it in the heat of battle as it were. Preferably we want to use this technique *at the exact time we start to focus on our tinnitus or to feel bad*. That's the sweet spot where this technique has the most effect.

But often we find ourselves already enveloped in focusing on our tinnitus or feeling bad. That's okay too. As soon as we notice we're caught, we interrupt it.

Here's another example of how this technique might work in action. Let's say you are going through your day. You begin to focus on or be bothered by your tinnitus. You notice that you are focusing on your tinnitus. First, you need to recognize that this is the moment when you can do something to massively affect your response to tinnitus. Be glad. This is the moment when you can make the most difference both now and long-term on your tinnitus. What you do during this time can make a marked impact on how tinnitus affects you. In your mind say to yourself something like, "Ahhh, got you, this is the time I can make change." Take advantage of it. This is the key time.

Then *force yourself* to do something to interrupt that pattern. Again, maybe you purposely walk differently, make a funny face, repeat some phrase to yourself, sing a few bars of a song, name a few presidents, think about what you had for dinner last night, imagine what the weather will be tomorrow, focus on a single letter on a portion of written text. Do a whole series of things no matter how bizarre, strange, out of the ordinary, funny or ridiculous, but do things to change your focus and to interrupt that pattern—anything—to keep that old tape from running.

Then, let's say you forget about your tinnitus for a few seconds, minutes, or longer. Then it begins to rear its head in your consciousness again. And then once again, you interrupt the pattern as soon as you become aware of it. And on it goes.

If you interrupt a pattern enough times, it won't run anymore.

Don't beat yourself up if you can't do this as much as you might like. When and if you can, do it. Try it and keep trying it even if it doesn't work perfectly every time. Each time you interrupt a negative response pattern or even try, it is like making a deposit into a bank account. The deposits begin to add up.

What about thinking about and worrying about tinnitus in the abstract? Why not interrupt that pattern too. Use the same methods above to avoid excessive thinking about and worrying about tinnitus. If you find yourself endlessly thinking, analyzing, evaluating your situation, then interrupt that habit too. The Nike slogan says, "Just Do It." Our slogan for tinnitus could be, "Just Don't Do It."

You now have a simple, down-and-dirty method for dealing

with tinnitus at least some of the time. In the next chapter, we will look a little more closely at what makes up our habits or patterns and further refine our techniques of interrupting negative tinnitus patterns.

Chapter Twelve

Disrupting Our Negative Patterns

In this chapter, we'll expand on the last chapter, and take a closer look at our habitual ways of responding to stimuli, our neuropathways, how this directly relates to tinnitus, and further bust-up and disrupt negative ways of responding to tinnitus.

We all create habits or patterns of responding to stimuli. Something happens to us, and we decide or create a certain way of dealing with it. Then, when that same stimulus happens again, we respond in the same manner. It's like a short cut. We do this in part to avoid having to deal with the same problem as an entirely new thing each time it occurs.

Some of the time these habits we create are beneficial; some of the time they are not.

Here's how a habit or pattern gets started. Imagine yourself walking across a field of waist-high grass. The first time you walk through the field, there is no path. You push your legs through the grass, and when you look back the way you came, you can see a faint path of bent-over grass. If you walk across that field again, there will be a tendency to follow that first faint pathway you made. This time you will press the grass down even more, and perhaps be able to see some actual soil underneath your feet. Over time it becomes only natural to keep walking down that same pathway when you cross the field. It's easy. Why create another path? This one is getting tamped down and is easy to follow. Less work. In fact, pretty soon no grass remains, and you are walking on a well-worn path. Eventually, our path can become a dirt road, then a paved road and maybe even a superhighway. This is analogous to what occurs in our brains. Habits (ways of responding) start off like that faint pathway across our field, but as we repeat them over and over, they become deeper and more ingrained. Just as our pathway across the field allows us to cross the field quickly, the neuropathways we develop in our brains allow us to respond quickly to stimuli and be whisked to an outcome as it were. Again, this is not all bad—it is just the way it is.

To carry the pathway analogy a bit further, the pathways we create can lead us to a good place, a bad place, or a neutral place. Given a choice (once we become aware of this), we want our pathways and their corresponding neuropathways in our brains to bring us to feeling neutral or good, but certainly not bad.

In the same way, we develop habitual ways of responding to tinnitus that lead us to feeling good, bad, or neutral. When we first got our tinnitus or perhaps at a time when it was particularly disturbing, we may have developed negative neuropathways that whisk us to a place of feeling bad. Again, this can become automatic. We experience the stimuli (hear our tinnitus), and we move quickly down our highway to our set response of feeling bad. This can occur seemingly almost without thinking and may seem beyond our control. We hear or focus on our tinnitus—we feel bad. We hear or focus on our tinnitus—we feel bad. Just like that. Every time. Same thing.

So what we want to do is first, become aware of our patterns, our habitual ways of responding to tinnitus, and then second, we want to take steps to destroy any negative patterns so they can't work anymore, so we can't follow them anymore. Finally, we want to create pathways that lead to us feeling neutral, good, or perhaps even empowered.

Using our pathway or road analogy again, first, we want to disrupt our old negative pathways so we can't follow them anymore. But we don't just want to throw a spadeful of dirt over our old negative pathways. We want to bulldoze the road so you can't drive on it anymore, we want to pile rocks so you can't get through, we want to dynamite ravines that can't be crossed, we want . . . well, you get the idea.

But before we do that, let's take a closer look at what makes up our patterns.

The bedrock of our patterns is our beliefs. That's why it's so important that you begin correcting and altering any non-resourceful beliefs as described in a previous chapter. Otherwise, one part of you will be pulling yourself in a new positive direction, while another part of you (your beliefs) will be saying, "This won't work," or "I can never get better." The methods that follow will still work, but they will work more efficiently if your beliefs are in sync with them.

The other two things that make up our patterns are the words and phrases we use in our self-talk and the way we move our bodies. We talked about the words and phrases we use in a previous chapter, so let's talk a little bit now about the physical aspects of our response patterns.

We Move and Position Our Bodies In a Certain Way When We Feel Bad

If we feel a certain way, we move a certain way. If we feel happy, we tend to move in an animated manner. We lift our heads and shoulders. We push out our chests. We smile. We move more quickly. We have more tone and life in our bodies. We talk faster and with more tonality in our voices. And when we feel down and depressed, we move differently. Our heads and shoulders drop. We droop. We look downward. We frown and wrinkle our brows. Our voices often become a monotone.

If you are feeling bad about tinnitus on a regular basis, invariably during the exact moments that you are feeling bad you are positioning and moving your body in a way that correlates with, creates, and maintains that feeling-bad emotion. These movements may be big and dramatic, or they may be subtle, but you are doing them.

Pick a time when you characteristically feel bad (overcome, discouraged, worried, angry, depressed, frustrated) about your tinnitus. How exactly do you position and move your body during those times? What exactly do you do with your body?

Here are some examples of the exact physical movements and positioning I would make when I felt bad about tinnitus.

When I was at my worst, I would lie on my stomach on the bed, close my eyes, put my face in a pillow, clasp both ears with my hands, and slowly rock forward and backward.

Another example—if I were sitting down and trying to do something and became overcome by the tinnitus, I would tilt my head to the left and downward, sigh, clasp my left ear, close my eyes, and drop my shoulders.

Or maybe it would be subtle; I'd just sigh and close my eyes.

All this detail may not seem important? But bear with me—it will be.

So what might be one example of the sequence of movements you characteristically do when you are feeling bad at a specific time about tinnitus? Write down one example for yourself. Be specific. What exactly do you do step by step? What exactly does it look like?

To help you do this exercise, imagine someone playing your part in a movie. You are the director. You want the actor to play your part perfectly. You need to explicitly tell them, for example, "First, you need to tilt your head downward, then you need to exhale deeply letting your shoulders fall, then while letting your shoulders fall, you need to shake your head slowly from side to side."

Have you got one of your physical sequences written down? Good.

Now we need to insert the sound track. We need to add anything we might say to ourselves (our self-talk) during the pattern we picked. Remember the negative self-talk we discussed in a previous chapter? What do you say to yourself when you feel bad? What tone do you use? Along with what you say, do you sigh, moan, or simply exhale?

For me, I'd say things to myself like, "I can't take this anymore," "God, I hate this," or "I'll never get better." And I'd say these things to myself with a distinctive depressed tonality.

Now I want you to insert your soundtrack, the words, phrases, and sounds you make, into the appropriate parts of your feeling-bad sequence.

So now, for me, I would have something like this—

I notice or focus on my tinnitus.
I tilt my head down and to the left.
I say to myself in a low, depressed voice, "God, I hate this."
I sigh deeply.

I clasp my left ear.
I drop my shoulders and lose most of the tone in my body.
I say to myself, "This will never go away."
I close my eyes.
I feel miserable.

Is it always exactly like that? No, but it's close enough. Have you written down a sequence for yourself delineating what you do with your body and say to yourself during a representative episode when you feel bad? Again, your movements may or may not be as dramatic as some of mine. Maybe you just tilt the corners of your mouth downward and sigh or say something like, "Here we go again."

Now let's put our sequences aside for a moment—

While most people understand that when we feel a certain way, we move a certain way, fewer people are aware that it works the other way as well. We can purposely make ourselves feel bad by moving in ways that mirror the way we move when we actually do feel bad. And we can make ourselves feel good or at least better by deliberately moving in ways that mirror positive emotions.

Try it. I want you to stand up, slump your shoulders forward, lower your chin and put a downcast, glum look on your face. Now, while maintaining all that, I want you to shuffle forward barely lifting your feet and scraping them along the floor as you walk. If you want—for added effect—you can mumble something like, "I feel so depressed. I am so depressed," as you shuffle forward.

Well, how did you start to feel? If you are like most people, you probably began to feel a little depressed and down by doing that. If you kept walking around like that, you would feel *very* depressed and ineffectual in a short time.

Now try it the other way. Stand up, throw your shoulders back, lift your head, smile, and walk around the room as if you were king or queen of the world. How do you feel?

You might begin to see where I'm going with this—what if we purposely replaced some of the steps in our negative sequence with the opposite (positive) physical movement and self-talk?

Here's how it might work for me in my example.

I notice or focus on my tinnitus.
I purposely lift my head up and look upward.
I say to myself in an enthusiastic voice, "Each day I'm getting better at handling this."
I smile.
I don't clasp my ear.
I raise my shoulders and chest.
I say to myself, "Each time I take any small action, the power this has over me diminishes."
I open my eyes wide.

And how do I feel? I feel neutral, or I even feel good. But I certainly don't feel bad and overcome by tinnitus.

What you are trying to do is to change steps in *your own personal specific* sequence on purpose. You are changing them from negative, feeling-bad movements and self-talk to positive, feeling-good ones.

Write down alterations for each of the steps in your sequence, changing each of them to positive steps.

Now I want you to purposely play-act your whole sequence in its new improved form. Act it out. Run through it several times with the new, positive steps inserted. How does it feel? How do you feel?

The way we use this technique is similar to our interrupting technique in the previous chapter. In the previous chapter, we simply interrupted things. In this chapter, we are fine tuning our attack and making it more directed.

Now, when we first notice—*when we get that first glimmer*—of going down one of our negative pathways, we consciously, purposely throw some or all of our positive steps into the mix. We purposely force ourselves to move and talk to ourselves using positive steps that we made up. It's important to note that this is not just a matter of talking and acting positive in any old way. Rather, we want to do it in a way that uses positive permutations of our old negative pattern. Not only are we not using our old negative pattern steps, but also we are specifically altering aspects of them to make them positive. This amplifies the effect of disrupting the old pattern.

Or we might find ourselves already stuck in a negative pathway. We might notice, "Hey, I've been feeling bad about this tinnitus for quite a while now." What do we do? We immediately act out and say to ourselves some of our positive steps.

Do you need to do all your steps? No, just enough or a few key ones to break your pattern. The idea is to throw in enough of the altered (positive) steps so that the pattern can't run the way it used to run. We don't want the old pattern to be able to complete itself, to play out, the way it used to. We don't want it to lead us to where it has been leading us in the past—to feeling bad.

Along with turning our negative steps into positive steps to disrupt a negative pathway, we can also simply make fun of the steps in our sequences. We can exaggerate our old steps or make them comical or simply bizarre. This serves the same purpose of disrupting the negative pattern.

Here's how this method might work for my example—

I notice or focus on my tinnitus.
I drop my head *way* down until it is almost touching the floor.
In a falsetto voice I say, "God, I hate this," making it sound ludicrous.
I pinch my left ear hard.
I inhale deeply and hold my breath puffing out my cheeks.
Then like a cartoon character, I ask, "Will this ever go away? Beats me!"

I've just disrupted the pattern. And how do I feel? I don't know how I feel. But again I have just prevented myself from going down my negative tinnitus pathway. Another way of thinking about it is that it is akin to putting snippets of aberrant code in a computer program. The program won't be able to run the way it used to run. Not only that, but I've also caused some long-term damage to the original sequence. I've just made it that much harder to play that sequence with all the conviction I used to have. Even it starts to run automatically sometimes, I might start thinking about the funny cartoon voice I used or allowing my head to drop all the way to the ground. I won't be able to feel the old sequence in the same way.

Sometimes the most absurd, silly, bizarre, and exaggerated interruptions of our sequences work best. You might think this is beneath you or too silly—but it works. No one needs to see or know what you're doing in private or in your mind if people are around. You also might feel uncomfortable making fun of yourself in this way. I'm not saying that your discomfort is not real. I'm not saying that you are not feeling bad. That's the exact reason we're doing this; that's the exact reason we *have to do this*—because we are feeling bad, and we want to change it. And remember, our goal is to do whatever it takes to limit the effect tinnitus has on our lives. If that means acting a little silly, it's worth it.

If you can use this technique once or a few times a day and it works, that is that many fewer times you weren't caught up in your tinnitus.

Finally, here's another thing you might try with your sequence. Change the order of some of the steps in your sequence. This also has the effect of not allowing our sequence to run to its negative completion. For one of your steps, draw an arrow and move that step to another location out of the usual sequence so it occurs where it shouldn't yet be occurring. If you first drop your shoulders and then emit a loud sigh and then say to yourself, "This is terrible," then change the order of those things. First say, "This is terrible," then sigh, then drop your shoulders. Try it for your original sequence—change some of the steps around. Or what if you decided just to pretend to feel bad first, and then do some of the preliminary steps that used to lead up to it.

Use whichever variation of these techniques work best for you. Mix and match. Disrupt your old feeling-bad sequences whenever you can, whenever you start to go down them, or whenever you find yourself in them. This process can also become more streamlined over time. After awhile when I just *began* to feel depressed or discouraged, when I just started to feel that first smidgen of beginning to focus on my tinnitus and feel overwhelmed, I could do one little thing like lift my head and smile and break the whole cycle of going down that negative path. And often, as a result, I would forget about the tinnitus and not focus on it anymore for a period of time

Again, what we want with this is to become incapable of running our old negative patterns in the way we used to. We want to interrupt our negative patterns as many times and in as many ways as we can.

Are there other times during the day when you characteristically feel bad about your tinnitus? Are there other situations when you characteristically feel bad? Write down some of those sequences. Now disrupt them first on paper by any of the above methods, and then act out the sequences in their altered forms.

To repeat, the best time to interrupt your patterns is at the exact moment they start to play. That is money. Don't wait. Play your new sequence or do something from your new repertoire right away.

The final thing we can do with our old—notice I'm already calling them "old"—tinnitus patterns is substitute steps that make us feel truly empowered into our sequence when we hear or notice our tinnitus. This is an advanced step, but I'm confident you're ready for it.

What if when you first began noticing and getting upset with your tinnitus, you didn't just do something positive, but you did something that made you feel great about yourself and your life? What if you did something that made you feel powerful?

What if hearing our tinnitus was a signal, a message, to feel stronger than usual? Let's try it.

In DNA recombinant therapy, scientists chemically snip open a section of DNA in an organism and insert another section of useful or beneficial DNA from another organism, perhaps a section that encodes for making insulin or growth hormone. That's what we want to do—insert some coding into our sequence that makes us feel empowered.

You may have explored some reasons your tinnitus *could* make you feel good back in the 'belief' section of this book.

We could feel good because having tinnitus is a message that life is short and we now need to live fully and make the most out of our lives and relationships. Tinnitus could remind us to live bigger and bolder than we may have otherwise. We could be inspired to take more chances perhaps and even do things we were postponing.

We could tell ourselves that if things such as tinnitus can happen in our lives, then we no longer need a reason to be happy. We no longer need to worry about stuff and can and should feel happy for no reason.

We could feel good because we know that at some level tinnitus is making us a stronger, better person, perhaps more compassionate, caring, and loving.

I'm going to use the first example—hearing my tinnitus empowers me to live my life to the fullest.

The first thing I want to do is think of movements that would embody "living life to the fullest" for me. I decide I'm going to lift my head, smile, and clench my right fist as if I just scored the winning point in a championship game. At the same time, I'm going to say, "Yes!" and "Hearing the ringing is a message to me that I'm going to live my life to the fullest." I can make this sequence shorter later, but this is what I'm going to do for now.

To embed this, I stand up—I want to be in an empowered state, I don't want to be slumping in some chair—and I listen for and find my tinnitus. The instant I focus on my tinnitus, I make my movements (lifting head, smiling, and clenching my right fist in a powerful, winning way) and say aloud or to myself, "Yes! Hearing this is a message to myself that I'm going to live my life to the fullest." The key here is to really feel what you are saying. I don't just want to go through the motions. I really do want to live life to the fullest, don't you? I want to show it. Feel it. For a few seconds, I want to capture that feeling inside myself that I truly am unstoppable and am going to live my life to the fullest no matter what my age or condition.

Then what do I do? I repeat the whole procedure lots of times. I listen for my tinnitus, make my movements, say my phrase, and feel empowered and strong. Listen for my tinnitus, make my movements, say my phrase, and feel empowered and strong. Listen for my tinnitus, make my movements, say my phrase, and feel empowered and strong. A dozen times is good.

Now it's your turn. Hearing your tinnitus is going to make you feel _____. What movement (s) are you going to make to reinforce this feeling in yourself? What word or phrase are you going to say? Do it. Give it a try. Remember, find your tinnitus for a second and then go into your new empowering pathway. Feel it. Find your tinnitus—go into your new empowering pathway. Repeat it a dozen times.

How about when you are walking or moving and notice your tinnitus? Perhaps, instead of feeling discouraged, that could trigger you to move and walk even more proudly or confidently.

What we are doing with this is disrupting our old patterns, and starting to embed a new reality into our psyches. We're telling ourselves that there is another possible way to think about our tinnitus and respond to it. Even doing this procedure a few times puts some scratches and disruptions into your old pattern. Part of you can't be quite as confident that tinnitus needs to be all bad.

Make up different movements and phrases you might say to yourself. After awhile, after reinforcing them enough times, you might not even need to go through the whole process. You can just hear your tinnitus and whoosh! You feel good and empowered. It can start to become automatic.

The Pattern Interrupter

What you are going to do here is make your very own Pattern Interrupter. Sounds like fun, doesn't it? Well, it is, and it will be.

And again, it's silly, but it works.

Get a piece of scrap paper and list all the different physical movements and things you might say to yourself when you feel bad with tinnitus. This will include steps from all your sequences. Use scissors and cut out these individual steps. Now write out distortions of each of the steps you cut out on another piece of paper. Make your distortions a combination of positive, bizarre, and empowering variations of your steps. For example, if I usually say to myself, "I can't take this anymore," I write "I can't fake this anymore." If I usually slump over, I write, "Get up and stamp your feet." You get the idea. Cut these out as individual commands also.

Now write down some random things for yourself to do that have nothing to do with tinnitus. Write each of these things down individually. Here are some examples: Think of a red brick; Get up and sweep a small section or the floor or think about sweeping the floor; Sing a few bars of James Brown's *I Feel Good*; Say the letters of the alphabet from 'L' to 'F' backwards; Imagine the taste of something sweet; Stand up and turn around once.

Now take all your separate slips of paper and put them in a jar or a ziplock bag. You've just created your very own Pattern Interrupter. Anytime you start to feel bad about your tinnitus, anytime you start to focus on your tinnitus in an unhealthy manner, simply pull out—let's say—three slips of paper and do what they say.

You may think I've gone overboard on this pattern-interrupting thing. But I can't emphasize it enough; the more times and ways you can stop the patterns of focusing on and feeling bad about tinnitus from occurring, the less of a hold tinnitus will have on you.

Chapter Thirteen

Scrambling Things Up (Even More)

The more we can scramble up our old or ineffective ways of looking at and dealing with tinnitus, the better. What we are doing is creating the space for our new beliefs to start to take hold, and for whatever other methods we are using to work. We want to shake things up. We want to create doubt in our minds about the way we used to think about tinnitus. We want to become a little confused about how we actually should view tinnitus, and thus create the space and become open to new alternative ways of looking at it. This chapter provides alternative—sometimes seemingly bizarre—techniques and ways of looking at tinnitus.

What if the way we are dealing with tinnitus is actually a game we are playing with ourselves?

Have you ever been doing something and then realized it was a game, and once you realized it was just a game, you couldn't take it seriously anymore? Let's say you were at work and your co-workers were playing a trick on you and you thought you had to get something done by a particular time. Then you realized it was a game and that they were just fooling around. Before you realized it was a game, you were serious. Once you realized they were up to their old shenanigans, you no longer took it seriously. What if we were playing a game with ourselves with regards our tinnitus?

The game is we think we have to feel bad about tinnitus. We think we should feel bad about tinnitus. We think it's reasonable, valid, sane, honest, authentic—real. After all, if so many people are disturbed about this, it must be valid, right? In fact, if someone told you it was a game you were playing all along, you would vehemently deny it and would say the exact opposite, "Nice try, but this really is real, and calling it a game won't change anything."

But what if at some level we are playing a game with this and then pretending that we aren't? How might you be playing a game with yourself with regards your tinnitus?

What if some of us were playing a game with ourselves that we couldn't win? That would be silly, wouldn't it? Think about that for a second. We have this ringing in our ears. By definition, we are going to hear it sometimes—after all, it is ringing in our ears! But then we set it up that when we hear it or notice it, we feel bad. Talk about a no-win situation.

Are there different ways to respond to tinnitus?

To borrow a story from Milton Erickson, the famed hypnotherapist, how many ways are there to enter a room? Well, you can enter through the door, through a window, dig a hole through the floor or ceiling. You could crawl in on your belly, or scurry in sideways like a crab. But you could also first fly to Amsterdam, then return via London and then stroll into the room. Or you could build the room around you.

The point is there are more ways of looking at things and solving things than we are aware of.

We often tend to think, "Well, everyone has thought of everything already. What could I possibly come up with?" Answer: You could come up with something that works for *you.* Brainstorm, have fun, be outrageous, play around with ideas, be imaginative. Often the silliest ideas have a spark of genius in them.

Write down in your notebook half a dozen ways new ways you might deal with your tinnitus. They don't have to make complete sense right now. Why might they work? How could you incorporate some of these ideas in the way you deal with tinnitus?

How about if everyone was born with tinnitus, would it still be a problem? Imagine that everyone you see has tinnitus. How would that make you feel?

Here's another idea—can we control how we respond to our tinnitus? Can we fake it? Can we be upset about our tinnitus at any given time and act like we're not? And conversely, can we not be upset, and act as if we are overwhelmed and severely depressed? How about trying that for a day. Every time you feel bad, act upbeat. Every time you feel good, purposely put on your depressed face and pretend you're sad and discouraged with your tinnitus. Is that fair? Or if you have someone you discuss your tinnitus with, when you feel bad, tell them you feel good and that the tinnitus is not bothering you, and when you feel good, tell them that the tinnitus is extremely bad and bothering you.

Why would we want to do this? To show ourselves, that we actually have more control over how we respond than we often acknowledge.

Here's another thing I'd like you to try—

I want you to change one small habit in some other area of your life completely unrelated to tinnitus. If you normally shave with a razor, use an electric razor. If you usually take your coffee black, start using a little creamer. Purposely change a small habit in *another* area of your life. Try it.

And if you have had tinnitus for a long time and are still bothered by it, try changing one little insignificant thing you do in your routine to handle it.

Here's another thing you can do—

If you characteristically feel bad about your tinnitus at a certain time of day or in a certain location, I want you to purposely feel bad about it at a different time of the day or at a different location. Force yourself to feel bad when you normally wouldn't.

Another thought—

What if you aren't the same person who was initially upset about tinnitus, or maybe the same person who started reading this book? What if you are not that person anymore, but you are still acting like that person, or think you need to act like that person. That person is *back there,* and you are here. I guess you wouldn't really need to keep acting like that person—of course, you could—but you wouldn't have to.

People also can change the way they react to things in their lives quickly or slowly. Which type of person do you think you are?

Maybe you are even trying to change and adjust to this tinnitus thing *too fast.* You might need to slow down. It won't do you any harm to stay the way you are a little longer. This tinnitus is a big deal, and you don't want to handle it too fast.

Or here is an idea—

Why not consolidate your time focusing on the ringing in your ears? You don't need to focus on it for fifty-five minutes every hour but for five minutes (use a timer) every hour, you are just to sit and listen to and focus on your tinnitus. No distractions. Don't do anything at the same time. Just listen and hang out with your tinnitus. Five minutes.

Or this—try the opposite. You can focus on your tinnitus for most of the day, but for five minutes every day, I want to you to make a conscious effort not to feel bad. Just five minutes.

Or you might decide that you will allow yourself to feel bad about this your tinnitus until a certain date and then stop.

Or you might just decide to put your tinnitus aside for now? Or you might decide that the attention and focus you give to tinnitus you might give to something else like getting your finances in order or preparing for the holidays.

Let's take a break from all this and just have some fun—

Our minds respond to images. It likes them. It lives off them. So let's have some fun with images. Imagine your tinnitus.

Watch your tinnitus being blown away.

Take a paintbrush, some paint and paint over your tinnitus until you can't see it anymore.

Take an eraser and erase its effects on you.

Imagine your tinnitus floating in water, and now drill holes into it until it sinks.

Dry it up.
Shoot it up.
Cut it up.
Pour chemicals over it and watch it dissolve.
Set it on fire.
Zap it.
Drive over it.
Sweep it up and throw it out.

Bomb it.
Exterminate it.
Forget about it and leave it behind somewhere.
Put it way off to the side and out of sight.

Or imagine your tinnitus as a funny little creature that you agree to live with in harmony. You've set boundaries for its behavior, but otherwise it can stay.

You know how you can super-size something. Well, downsize your tinnitus. Imagine it going from gargantuan to big to medium-sized then finally to tiny and disappearing altogether.

Or maybe you want to put your tinnitus in a large manila envelope and store it somewhere. When you want to worry about it, take the envelope out and worry about it. When you are done, put the envelope away.

Now you make up a few.

Finally, in the spirit of this chapter, I'd like to suggest how long it will take—and this is only a suggestion—for you to start feeling results from doing the things in this book. Maybe it will occur no sooner than in one day but no longer than in two and a half weeks.

Chapter Fourteen

Make It a Game

Despite what I may have said in an earlier chapter, we all like games. Games are fun. We don't take them as seriously. You score points. Maybe you progress around a board or get a ball in a hole. You win prizes. Often we do better at something if we make it fun, if we enjoy the process.

If I tell you in my best doctor voice that I want you to consistently attempt to cognitively change the way you represent tinnitus to yourself, it sounds pretty dull and boring. No fun. It sounds like a job or a chore. You probably wouldn't want to do it.

But if I told you it's really a game you can play with your tinnitus on a daily basis, you might go, "Hmmm, that sounds interesting and fun."

Now the rules of this game are a bit strange in that they are only to your benefit (since you are the only player). You can *only* receive points; you can't lose points. You can only get points, but how many points you get is up to you.

You get a point or score anytime you handle your tinnitus in any way that keeps it from bothering you. For example, anytime you use any of the techniques in this book to squelch your tinnitus from distracting you or depressing you, you get points.

Let's say your tinnitus starts to bother you, and you smoothly, efficiently put on some music. You don't get overly involved in thinking about your tinnitus. You don't think about tinnitus. You just put on music. You just do it. That's worth points.

Or let's say you just start, just barely start for a few microseconds, to listen and obsess about your tinnitus such that it starts to bother you. But instead of falling into that trap, you interrupt things using any of the techniques in the previous chapters—you get points. "Gotcha," you might say to yourself, as you rack up the points.

Maybe your tinnitus is going to stop you from doing something, but instead, you decide to do that thing anyway, in spite of your tinnitus. Unless absolutely necessary, you are not going to let tinnitus limit what you do. More points.

You read, reread, or practice any of the techniques in this book—major bonus points.

You can also get bonus points if you use one of the methods in this book in a particularly novel or imaginative way. For example, if you start to get overwhelmed by your tinnitus, and you got up and danced a little jig to interrupt the pattern, then that would be worth bonus points for sure.

Depending on your situation, if you need masking sound to go to sleep, and you try—just try—for a minute or so to sleep without sound, give yourself a few points. Depending on your situation, if you try not to take a pill for your tinnitus and just try to get by, that might be worth a few points.

Or maybe you have a particularly bad day with your tinnitus, and you *don't* dwell on it but simply move on. Or you feel bad and you do one simple tiny thing different (better) in dealing with your tinnitus. You just do one simple thing. You try even once. Well, that's worth a lot of points because you were under a lot of strain, and it may have taken great effort to take even any small step.

Maybe one time, instead of thinking negatively about tinnitus, you remember one of your beliefs that perhaps tinnitus could somehow make you a better person or to live more fully in the ways that you can. You just scored points.

What are some other ways you might award yourself points specific to your own personal situation?

Again, there's no way you can lose this game. You might even imagine a large brightly-lit, blinking scoreboard with casino-type, slot-machine-type jangling bells compounding your winnings, as you go through your day.

Chapter Fifteen

Action Plan

Now is the time to put all the pieces we've developed into an action plan.

First—

Did you get a complete workup for your tinnitus as recommended? If not, do not collect $200, do not pass go. Get a complete, thorough workup for your tinnitus *now*.

Are you aware of the various therapies for tinnitus? Are you using some of them? Again, the methods in this book work in conjunction with whatever else you are doing to deal with your tinnitus.

Do you recognize that you probably have to go through a period of feeling bad (the five stages) about your tinnitus before you can fully start working on it? Accept that fact—it's normal and okay.

The central premise of this book is that dealing with tinnitus is in great part a mental endeavor. We want to use our minds to be on our side in dealing with tinnitus.

Remember our rules—

This can and will change for the better.

Any little thing we do, even once, that moves us in the direction of controlling our mind helps and makes a difference. These little steps we take begin to add up and have a cumulative effect.

Let's review some of the aspects of this book. Do you have strong enough reasons for why you absolutely, positively must handle this? Have you decided? Have you made up your mind that you've had enough and you are going to handle this? Nothing is going to stop you. Do you feel you must handle this? Are you aware of the costs if you don't? If not, go back and reread the chapter on motivation. Motivate yourself.

Have you developed a series of strong new beliefs about tinnitus, the main one being that you can have tinnitus, you can hear ringing in your ears, but you don't have to be upset, mad, angry, overcome, or depressed because of it. Have you written down your new beliefs and have you started reinforcing them and *feeling* them perhaps on a daily basis. Are your new beliefs starting to become you?

Are you trying to ask better questions about yourself? Remember, the questions we ask ourselves in great part determine how we view tinnitus, and hence, how it affects us.

What about the words you use? Have you become conscious of how the words and phrases you use affect how you represent tinnitus to yourself and the effect it has on you? Have you changed some of the words and phrases you use?

Have you started to interrupt your negative neuropathway habits in simple ways or by using altered elements of your own specific pathways? Are you interrupting the times you focus too much on your tinnitus or feel bad on a regular basis, or as much as you can at this time? Have you tried to substitute some positive empowering feelings for your old negative ones?

You can't always know which of the techniques in this book will work best for you, or in what combination. That's why I encourage you to experiment with all of them. Often, one little thing, one new way of looking or dealing with tinnitus can 'click' and produce dramatic improvements in the way you deal with tinnitus.

Also, give yourself time. It sometimes takes time for our bodies and minds to integrate things.

What else can you do?

How about setting aside some time each day to work on changing your mind about tinnitus, to reinforce the principles and methods in this book. Maybe you can commit a few minutes every morning to getting your mind straight about tinnitus before your day gets started. Make it a habit.

Perhaps sit down and go over one aspect of this book or some of your notes on what you've discovered and figured out for yourself. You could go over your new beliefs. Remember the key to the reaffirming the new beliefs is to actually *feel* each one in your body for a few seconds.

Maybe work on some of the questions you've developed to ask yourself or try to come up with new questions and even more-empowering answers. Maybe practice some of the techniques of interrupting your pattern in case you go into a slump or feel overwhelmed during the day. Plan for what your day is going to be like for you, and how you are going to handle things with regards your tinnitus today. What strategies will you use?

My strategy was to keep hammering away at tinnitus by constantly reinforcing my positive beliefs and reinforcing every action I took, no matter how small, to disrupt any patterns of feeling bad. Tinnitus can't stand a chance over the long run. For me—when I was at my worst—it was necessary and worthwhile to commit some serious time to this process every day. That's how we get good at something. Practice makes permanent.

Along with this, please do remember to be grateful for all that you do have. No matter how bad our lives can seem at any instant, there are always things we can be thankful for. And be especially loving and appreciative of yourself. You *are* taking specific actions to handle tinnitus. It can be a hard thing to do. You are teaching your mind that you will not accept allowing it to overwhelm you or make you depressed or discouraged. Whether you feel it or not at any given instant, trust me, you are making progress.

Again, reinforce and encourage yourself for the action you *are* taking. Congratulate yourself.

Keep a Log

The next thing I would suggest is that you keep a log. Keep a written record of how your tinnitus affects you at various times of the day, and try to discern any factors that make it better or worse. Write down how good or bad you would rate your tinnitus and your response to it. No need for graphic details on how bad it might be. Just write down your observations in a matter-of-fact manner like a scientist. Write down the actual times when you take a reading of your tinnitus. How loud is it when you wake up in the morning? How loud in the afternoon? What time did you wake up, and what did you eat or drink in the morning? And at what times? Does anything you do make a difference in the perceived loudness, or its effect on you?

Become curious. Be open to whatever insights you might gain by doing this. Try to discover patterns. Don't presume to know all the answers no matter how long you've had tinnitus.

What if—just by being curious—you could discover something for yourself that makes a big difference in diminishing the intensity of your tinnitus?

How can you experiment or incorporate what you discover into your overall tinnitus plan?

For example, as you may be aware, common factors that may or may not exacerbate tinnitus in a given individual include such things as stress of any kind, sleep deprivation, hydration status, salt intake, alcohol, caffeine to name just a few. In keeping with the theme of this book, we want to do all we can on every front to handle our tinnitus. If you could find ways to do this by keeping a log and recording your observations, then that would most assuredly be worthwhile.

What about experimenting with some of the different adjuncts for tinnitus. If you use earplugs in noisy environments, perhaps experiment with different types. If you use music to help mask your tinnitus, what type of music works the best. Take action. Don't be helpless. Do what you can to find ways that make things better. Along with controlling our minds, we want to have as many variables as possible be in our favor.

Also, in your log, record your progress. Write down your successes. Remember one of our other rules: We only tend to be aware of the times we are bothered by our tinnitus, not all the times we are not. Become aware of the times you interrupted a pattern, or how you may have prevented yourself from spiraling downward.

Stress - The Feedback Loop

There is a physiologically proven feedback loop for people with chronic pain. Stress causes their pain to get worse, and their pain getting worse causes more stress . . . which causes more pain. Round and round the circle it goes. It's like one of those Chinese finger traps—the harder you pull, the more you stay stuck. Sometimes we have to recognize that we have to consciously take actions to relieve our stress in order to decrease the hold tinnitus may have on us.

It can be the same thing with our tinnitus. Any form of stress (being dehydrated, hungry, tired, overworked, etc.) can cause our tinnitus to be perceived as louder and more invasive. This make us feel worse—to feel more stressed.

So anytime you can do anything to decrease your overall stress level or your stress over the tinnitus in particular, it is going to help. It is like being aware of a regulator knob that you have some control over.

What are some stressors in your life that make your tinnitus worse?

What can you do to alleviate those or diminish their effect? Write down specific small things you might do to manage your overall stress level. Take action to limit stress that exacerbates your tinnitus.

Sleeping

Sleeping can be a problem with tinnitus. For whatever reason often later in the day and at bedtime, tinnitus can get louder or more intrusive for many people. In part, this is because when we lie down to sleep, suddenly there is no ambient noise. We are left alone with silence . . . and our tinnitus. Many a time I remember laying my head on the pillow and hearing the roaring in my ear and thinking how could I ever fall asleep. And on many nights it was a real battle.

I'm sure you are aware of good sleep habits: go to bed at a set time, avoid stimulation before bedtime, don't drink caffeine or alcohol, try to get some exercise each day, use your bed and bedroom just for sleeping, don't use electronics before bedtime, use relaxation or meditation techniques. These are all good as far as they go, but they don't specifically address tinnitus.

The key to sleeping with tinnitus is to *have a plan*. Don't let going to sleep with tinnitus become a "thing." Don't allow it to become an ordeal for yourself. Have a plan in place in advance. Be matter of fact, practical. Say, "If this happens, I'm going to do this. Then if this happens, I'm going to do this." Practical step-by-step.

You may already have a plan or system you use if you have trouble going to sleep with tinnitus. Perhaps you play background music or some sort of white noise. But if you still are having problems, consider coming up with a more detailed, sequential plan.

Here was one plan I used for my tinnitus when I was at my worst.

First, I would make sure I would get into bed at the same time every night. Then I would always try to fall asleep for fifteen minutes without doing anything just as I had in the past before tinnitus. I wanted to start to re-educate myself that I could fall asleep without any help. However, if after fifteen minutes, I couldn't fall asleep, then I would go on to step two. I would put on my masking music next to my bed. Another twenty minutes and if I still hadn't fallen asleep, I take a tiny nibble of a sleeping pill, and continue with the masking music.

Sleeping pills are obviously a two-edged sword. My advice is if you need them, take them, particularly if you are going through a bad time with your tinnitus. They can be a godsend. They can give you that much-needed sleep and prevent sleep deprivation from compounded your dealing with tinnitus.

The downside to sleeping pills is that you can become dependent on taking sleeping pills both mentally and physiologically. We don't want that if we can avoid it. Many of these groups of medications generally produce some sort of dependence, again, either physiologically or mentally, and also have rebound and withdrawal phenomenon. When you stop using them after using them on a regular basis, it can be *very* difficult to fall asleep. For sedative type drugs, withdrawal symptoms are often the opposite of the sedative effect. That is, if you stop taking them after taking them for days in a row, you feel excessively agitated. I assume that most people reading this book don't want to become dependent on taking sleeping pills or anti-anxiety agents all the time. Use your judgment.

So putting it all together, if tinnitus is markedly disrupting your sleep, perhaps see your doctor and get something to help you to sleep. When other methods to fall asleep fail, use the pills. Take the smallest amount necessary. This means, depending on your individual dosage, you can cut the pills in half or into even smaller portions.

Even if you don't use them on a regular basis, just knowing you have these pills can help. You'll know in a pinch if it gets bad enough, you can take a pill and escape things at least for now. Just knowing that option is available would often help me to fall asleep when I was at my worst.

Make up a plan for sleeping. Follow it. I know it can be hard but try to avoid making a big deal out of sleeping.

Have a Plan For If Your Tinnitus Gets Bad

Just as we want to have a plan for sleeping, we want to have a plan for when and if our tinnitus gets bad. For whatever reason, at some times our tinnitus may seem more overwhelming or just plain louder. What are you going to do?

What are you going to do when you feel nothing you are doing is working, and you are beginning to feel overcome by your tinnitus? Or maybe you even feel that way now.

We have to have a plan.

First—and this is a big point—we have to expect that this might happen. Be ready for it. Be ready to say, "For whatever reason, I'm focusing on the ringing too much and feeling bad. My techniques of dealing with it aren't working as well as they might." That's okay. Remember the chapter when I said don't make a big deal out of it. Do what you need to do and move on. We also have to be aware that we make progress in handling our tinnitus often in a hurdy-gurdy, jerky manner. It is not always smooth or linear. We can do well for a few days and then seem to have a setback. Notice I say *seem* to have a setback. It is not really a setback because everything we've done and are doing is still working.

If you start to feel completely overcome, first I want you to be loving to yourself. This tinnitus can be a trying ordeal. You *are* being brave and strong trying to handle this. Cut yourself a little slack. Pat yourself on the back for all that you have done, and give yourself a little break.

Maybe you're just overly tired, or some unknown thing (we don't know all the causes of what makes tinnitus worse) is just causing the tinnitus to get worse, or something is causing your physiology to react this way.

Again, do whatever it takes at this point to handle the tinnitus.

Listen to masking music if that works for you. Take a pill to calm you down or to sleep. Do whatever it takes for you not to feel overwhelmed. The point is to have a plan in advance. Don't make a big deal out of it.

Do you remember that children's game called Red Light, Green Light? It is sometimes a bit like that with tinnitus. When you feel good, make as much progress as you can in dealing with tinnitus. When you feel bad, you might have to stand still.

Again, the things we put into effect through this book (and the other methods you may be using) may take some time to have their full effect. It is as if we have cast our lines and nets into the sea and we just have to wait for a period of time. We may not be aware of what is going on under the surface. Parts of our brain are integrating all the methods in this book; trust that they will work even if you may not feel it sometimes.

Sometimes this will even be a sort of last hurrah from your tinnitus, a last attempt to try and exert its dominance over you. If you can stay calm now, and do a few simple things, the payoff will be huge. If you can't or don't want to right now, that's okay too. Again, be loving to yourself.

The People in Your Life

When I first developed tinnitus, I thought—mistakenly—that my wife would appreciate frequent, almost-hourly updates on my tinnitus and my reactions to it. Well, as you might guess, even such a gentle soul as my wife quickly became bored and annoyed with my constant updates. How are you going to relate to the people in your life with regards your tinnitus?

It's safe to say people are concerned and interested . . . but only so much. We all like it when we see people taking action to solve their problems. Send a message to those around you that you may be upset and hurting sometimes but you are doing all in your power to get better and handle this.

Think about what is the best way, despite your tinnitus, for you to interact with the people in your life. How are you going to relate to people at home and work with regards your tinnitus? Decide.

Make It A Habit

All the methods in this book revolve around the principle that the more we consistently do something on a regular basis, the more it automatically, almost effortlessly, leads us to the desired goal.

All things being equal, a runner who makes it a habit of waking up every morning at 6 AM and running five miles will become a better runner. A salesperson who commits to making a given number of cold calls every day will have more sales.

Anything that we can commit to and make a habit we *will* get better at. So what are some of the things we can do to make habits out of the principles and techniques in this book? To reiterate, first we have to have clear motivation for why we are doing this; hopefully, you've developed this from the "Why" chapter. We don't want to sort-of-maybe-I-might-coulda-woulda try the things in this book. We want to *commit* to doing them. The next thing we want to do is not to start too big. For example, we don't want to demand from ourselves that we are immediately able to interrupt each and every time that we feel bad about tinnitus. We want to start small, and then slowly build. We want to feel encouraged, and support ourselves for any small steps we take in the right direction, again.

Another thing we might do is to design our environment in such a way that it reinforces our doing these things. That might mean putting up little notes for ourselves, or having our Pattern Interrupter readily available, or changing some aspect of our daily routine so that we have a regular set time to reinforce the principles in this book.

It's our consistent action that will make the methods in this book work, not doing things once in awhile and saying, "Oh, this doesn't work."

We want to make our new ways of dealing with tinnitus into habits. What are some things you could do to make both the principles and the methods in this book habits in your life?

Refining Our Technique

We are all different, and several times throughout this book I've said that we all individually know more than we suspect on how to handle tinnitus. The techniques in this book aren't written in stone.

By now, you should understand the general principle of this book—doing everything we possibly can to put our minds on our side in our interaction with tinnitus.

For every technique or principle in this book, you need to be constantly thinking how can I make this work better *for me*. Is there a slight variation to this method that might really work better for me? Try things. Experiment.

Being flexible in our dealing with tinnitus is to our advantage. The smart person is the one who, at regular intervals, assesses the effectiveness of what he or she is doing. Then, based on that evaluation, refines and improves his or her technique or strategy.

If at first, you don't succeed, keep trying but also be open to trying different things or modifying your approach slightly.

How can you modify some of the things in this book so that they work optimally for you?

Reinforcement

Reinforcement is an accelerant to accomplishing whatever we decide to do. Anytime we reinforce positive behavior, we get more of it. So if we want to make maximal progress in this process of handling tinnitus, we have to reinforce ourselves *for what we are doing* as much and as often as possible.

We want to reinforce ourselves for any little thing that we do. We want to reinforce ourselves for any tiny step we take, for any time when we might have been overwhelmed or discouraged with our tinnitus, but we interrupted that pattern and stepped out of there. Any one time. Any little time.

We want to recognize that we have the courage and gumption to want to handle this, and that we aren't just sitting on our bottoms being helpless victims. Instead, we are doing something.

How do we reinforce ourselves? Well, the easiest way is just to give ourselves a mental pat on the back anytime we move in the right direction. If you interrupt your tendency to be depressed by your tinnitus for a few seconds, tell yourself in your head, "Way to go!" If you remember one of your new beliefs and substitute it when an old belief comes up to haunt you, tell yourself, "That's it. I'm really doing this."

When is the best time to reward yourself and make yourself

feel good for what you *are* doing? Right away—the moment you do something to disrupt your old way of dealing with tinnitus. That is the moment when reinforcement and self-encouragement are most effective.

If you want you can even give yourself a reward of some sort for making progress over a number of days. Buy yourself your favorite food or something you like. You want to give yourself the message that you are going to reward yourself and feel good whenever you take steps—again, no matter how small—in the right direction.

What Has Worked Best For Me

While this book has been instructional, it has also been, in part, a personal chronicle of the methods I have used in dealing with tinnitus.

Hence, I feel it may be worthwhile to share some of the methods and principles that have worked best for me.

In no specific order—

- The idea of not *fighting* tinnitus.

- Not giving it energy.

- Becoming aware of the words I was saying.

- The idea of not being afraid to hear the ringing and not having to run and cover it every time I noticed it.

- The breaking of the connection that when I notice or hear my tinnitus that I *have to* feel upset, angry, or depressed.

- The changing of my beliefs. In particular, for me, it helped to think that this was a wake-up call, that because of having tinnitus, I could be spurred to living my life to the fullest.

- Consistently, interrupting my patterns whenever I began to feel bad.

- Remembering and reinforcing myself for taking small steps.

- Making strategies in advance on how I would deal with trying situations. Dealing with things in a matter-of-fact manner.

- Not dwelling on any setbacks but simply moving on.

- Spending time on a regular basis every morning developing and working on all the methods in this book.

Now it's your turn. What has worked best for you so far? What is your action plan for the future? Write it down. Commit to it. Take some time doing this. By now, you know that you can and will make progress. Do it.

Chapter Sixteen

Final Thoughts

Hopefully, after working your way through this book, the way you view tinnitus has changed. You don't look at tinnitus quite the same anymore.

You don't see yourself as a victim. You don't see yourself as someone stuck with an affliction, but rather as someone continually smoothly, efficiently addressing tinnitus both through standard treatment modalities and through the management of your mental state.

Our tinnitus may or may not go away. It may or may not diminish in intensity. It may, indeed, be something we are stuck with the rest of our lives. It doesn't matter. We will keep taking consistent steps to diminish its effect on us.

By now, you recognize that you play a very active role in both how you respond to tinnitus and to how it affects your life. That is both sobering and reassuring. You can no longer pretend to have absolutely nothing to do with tinnitus' effect on you, while at the same time you know that there are things only *you* can do to control your mental state and thus diminish tinnitus' effect on you.

You've been exposed to a number of techniques in this book; they all work but some may work better than others for you. But also remember that there is a cumulative, synergistic effect to the techniques. The more different ways you change your mind with regards tinnitus, the greater and quicker the results.

Some of these techniques can work right away to limit the effect tinnitus has on you in a given moment, but others, such as the new beliefs, may take some time to take hold fully.

All this requires your full strength and commitment. Put in the time and effort to make these new ways of thinking and techniques become habits, not just something you read about. Remember in the strategy chapter about setting aside some time each day to refine and perfect these techniques for yourself.

Maybe sometimes now you even forget for long periods of time that you have tinnitus. You may notice it's there, but you don't react. Or if someone asks you how you feel about it, you may not be quite sure anymore. You just don't think about it or focus on it as much anymore. Those are the ways to measure your progress.

Reward and reinforce your success every step of the way no matter how small it may seem. Small streams *do* grow into mighty rivers. You can and will master this.

You are worth it. No matter what your age, you still have a lot of life to live. Don't allow something both as disturbing yet as silly as tinnitus to ruin your life in any way.

About the Author:

Paul D'Arezzo, M.D. has worked for many years as a board-certified emergency physician. After developing severe tinnitus himself and desperately searching for a cure, he recognized the need to control his mind in dealing with tinnitus. The relative lack of readily-available materials on the mental aspects of tinnitus led him to craft a method, based on sound therapeutic principles, to diminish the effect tinnitus has on our lives.

Dr. D'Arezzo is the author of two previous books, *Posture Alignment* and *Functional Fitness*, both recently rewritten and republished as e-books under the titles *How To Improve Your Posture* and *Stay Active Longer*.

Made in the USA
Middletown, DE
17 August 2019